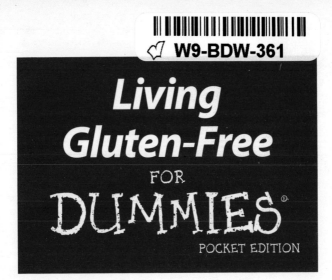

Living
Gluten-Free
FOR
DUMMIES®
POCKET EDITION

by Danna Korn

WILEY

Wiley Publishing, Inc.

Living Gluten-Free For Dummies®, Pocket Edition

Published by
Wiley Publishing, Inc.
111 River St.
Hoboken, NJ 07030-5774
www.wiley.com

Copyright © 2011 by Wiley Publishing, Inc., Indianapolis, Indiana

Published by Wiley Publishing, Inc., Indianapolis, Indiana

Published simultaneously in Canada

For general information on our other products and services, please contact our Customer Care Department within the U.S. at 877-762-2974, outside the U.S. at 317-572-3993, or fax 317-572-4002.

For technical support, please visit www.wiley.com/techsupport.

Wiley also publishes its books in a variety of electronic formats. Some content that appears in print may not be available in electronic books.

ISBN: 978-1-118-01404-2

Manufactured in the United States of America

10 9 8 7 6 5 4 3 2 1

WILEY

Table of Contents

. . . .

Introduction

. . . .

*N*ot so many years ago, the gluten-free lifestyle
was reserved for an obscure cluster of people
who were forced to settle for wannabe foods that
resembled sawdust but didn't taste as good.

Today, the gluten-free lifestyle is sweeping the world
with the force of a really big blowtorch, and the rami-
fications are enormous. Gluten-free products abound
(and are a far cry from the foods we used to choke
down), labels are far less ambiguous, and people no
longer look at you like you have four heads when you
ask for a burger without the bun.

Being gluten-free isn't about being on a diet. It's about
living a lifestyle. Whether you've been gluten-free for
decades or are only considering the idea of giving up
gluten, this book is loaded with information that can
affect every aspect of your life, from your health and
your bank account to your shopping, cooking, and
eating habits.

I live a gluten-free lifestyle, and I have for years. I have
no ulterior motives, other than some quirky desire to
don a cape, call myself the Glutenator, and travel far
and wide to extol the virtues of a gluten-free diet. I
have no supplements to sell you and no gluten-free
food products that I endorse. What matters to me is
that I do my best to tell you what you need to know
about living a gluten-free lifestyle so you can make
healthy decisions. That's why I've made this book
your reference guide for living — and loving — a
gluten-free lifestyle.

About This Book

This guide offers clear guidance on how to make the transition to a gluten-free lifestyle. And like all *For Dummies* books, this one is divided up so you don't have to read it all at once, or even front to back, if you don't want to. You can skip from B to R to A and even reread B if you want. You can read it sideways and standing on your head, if you'd like; all you have to do is find a section of interest to you and dig in (how's *that* for liberating?).

Conventions Used in This Book

I make up words, but they're pretty easy to figure out. For instance, *glutenated* means a product has been contaminated with gluten, *glutenous* means it has gluten in it, a *glutenivore* is something that eats gluten, a *Glutenator* is one who battles the evils of gluten, and so on. It's fun! In fact, I bet you'll soon be making up your own glutenologisms.

Here are some conventions that are specific to the recipes in Chapter 7:

- ✔ If an ingredient appears in a recipe, it's assumed to be gluten-free. For instance, I don't specify "gluten-free vanilla" because all vanilla is gluten-free. And soy sauce usually has gluten, but when I call for soy sauce in a recipe, I'm assuming you'll use a gluten-free version.

- ✔ Baking with gluten-free flours works best if you use a mixture of flours. (Chapter 5 goes into detail about how to mix gluten-free flours to get the best results.)

- ✔ Milk substitutes can be used in place of milk in most recipes.

✔ Eggs are large.

✔ Butter and margarine are interchangeable.

✔ All temperatures are in Fahrenheit.

Foolish Assumptions

You spent your hard-earned cashola on this book, which I'm guessing means you want to find out more about the gluten-free lifestyle. Well, good news! I've written this book with you in mind — and I've taken the liberty of making a few assumptions about you:

✔ You're considering going gluten-free and plan on using this book to determine whether to take the plunge.

✔ You love someone who's gluten-free, and you're so cool that you want to find out more about the lifestyle so you can be supportive.

✔ You're new to the diet and are looking for the "manual" that can tell you how to live a gluten-free lifestyle.

✔ You've been gluten-free for years and want the latest, greatest information about dietary guidelines and state-of-the-art research.

Icons Used in This Book

Some people are more visual than others. That's why icons are cool. This book uses several icons, and each one has a little tidbit of information associated with it. Here's what each icon means:

Everyone can use a friendly little reminder. The Remember icon is a quick and easy way to identify some of the more important points that you may want to make note of throughout the book.

Cleverly designated as Tips, these are, well, *tips* that can help you live (and love!) the gluten-free lifestyle. They include info to help you save time or cut down on frustration.

Text flagged with the Warning icon can keep you out of trouble.

Where to Go from Here

Curl up in your comfiest chair and dive right into the chapter or section that interests you most. Although if you're new to the gluten-free lifestyle and have tons of questions, you're probably best off starting at Chapter 1 and working your way through the book in order. Been gluten-free for years? Do yourself a favor and take a look at Chapter 3. You may be surprised by some of the foods now allowed on the gluten-free diet that used to be considered no-nos.

For even more information on living the gluten-free lifestyle, from details on celiac disease and how gluten affects behavior to advice on raising gluten-free kids, pick up the full-size version of *Living Gluten-Free For Dummies,* 2nd Edition (Wiley), available at your local bookstore or at www.dummies.com.

Finally, if you're feeling a little down about going gluten-free, I hope my sincere passion for the gluten-free lifestyle and the healthy benefits that go along with it touch you by offering comfort, optimism, and inspiration.

Chapter 1

Living Gluten-Free, From A to Z

. . . .

In This Chapter

▶ Getting a grip on gluten

▶ Discovering the pros of the gluten-free lifestyle

▶ Making the most of meals

▶ Loving going from gluten-gorger to gluten-free forager

. . . .

I figured the doctor had made a mistake. "You mean *glucose*," I corrected him with a tinge of exasperation at his clumsy blunder. "You must mean my son can't eat *glucose*." Geesh. This was going to be tough. No more gummi bears.

"No, I mean *gluten*," he insisted. "And to be honest, I really don't know much about the gluten-free diet. You can see our hospital dietitian, but she won't have much on the diet, either. You're going to have to do some homework on your own."

All I could muster was a blank stare. What the heck was *gluten*? Keep in mind the year was 1991, when I knew as much about gluten as I know about piezo-electric polymers. Approximately nothing.

Stranded on some figurative island located somewhere between Terror Bay and the Dread Sea, I figured I had two options: Tyler could starve to death, or I could get busy trying to figure out what the heck gluten was all about. Al Gore hadn't invented the Internet yet, and I couldn't find any books or support groups; it was time to get resourceful and creative. I was determined to find out everything I could — and then share it with the world (at least, the other six people on the planet who were gluten-free at the time).

Little did I know that gluten-free-ness would explode into what it is today — one of the fastest-growing nutritional movements in the world — and this mission of mine would become all-consuming. This chapter gives you a basic rundown of what living gluten-free is all about.

What Is Gluten, Anyway, and Where Is It?

Gluten has a couple definitions. One is technically correct but not commonly used; the other is commonly used but not technically correct. I give you more details on both definitions in Chapter 3, but to get you started, and for the purposes of most of this book, here's the common definition: *Gluten* is a mixture of proteins in wheat, rye, and barley. Oats don't have gluten but may be contaminated, so they're forbidden on a strict gluten-free diet, too.

You can find lots of information about what you can and can't eat in Chapter 3 and at www.celiac.com. But you need to have a general idea of what kinds of foods have gluten in them so you know what to avoid. Foods with flour in them (white or wheat) are the most common culprits when you're avoiding gluten. The following are obvious gluten-glomming foods:

- ✔ Bagels
- ✔ Beer
- ✔ Bread
- ✔ Cookies, cakes, and most other baked goods
- ✔ Crackers
- ✔ Pasta
- ✔ Pizza
- ✔ Pretzels

But along with these culprits come not-so-obvious suspects, too, such as licorice, most cereals, and natural flavorings. When you're gluten-free, you get used to reading labels, calling manufacturers, and digging a little deeper to know for sure what you can and can't eat.

You have to do without those foods, but you really don't have to do *without*. There's a subtle but encouraging difference because food manufacturers make delicious gluten-free versions of just about every food imaginable these days.

But I Thought Wheat Was Good for Me!

You may see lots of labels proudly declaring products to be wheat-free (some of which, like spelt and kamut, aren't really wheat-free at all). When something says it's wheat-free, it doesn't mean the food is gluten-free.

 Gluten is in wheat, but it's also in rye and barley — and most people don't eat oats on the gluten-free diet, either. So something can be wheat-free but still have other gluten-containing ingredients, such as malt, which is usually derived from barley. In that case, the product is wheat-free but not gluten-free.

Anyone who's spent more than a day on planet Earth has been barraged with messages hailing the virtues of wheat — especially in its whole form. Wheat and other grains hog most of the food pyramid(s), suggesting you should eat gobs of it, and it's touted as a good source of fiber and nutrients. Wheat does provide some health benefits, but you can find these benefits in other food sources, too. So how can wheat be at the root of so many health problems?

For three reasons, wheat may not be the key to perfect dietary health:

✔ **Wheat was invented yesterday.** Wheat wasn't introduced until the Agricultural Revolution, about 10,000 years ago — that's yesterday, evolutionarily speaking. Before that, people ate lean meats, fish, seafood, nonstarchy vegetables, berries, and fruits. When wheat came on the scene, it was completely foreign.

✔ **Humans don't fully digest wheat.** Human bodies have to adapt in order to tolerate wheat, and lots of people don't tolerate it well at all. Most humans have only one stomach — and one just isn't enough to digest wheat. Cows have four stomachs (actually, four chambers within one stomach). That's why Bessie the Bovine does okay with wheat. The wheat goes from one stomach to another and another and — well, you get the picture. By the time it reaches tummy number four, it's fully digested and Bessie's feeling fine.

✔ **Wheat contributes to leaky gut (*Z* is for *zonulin*).** When people eat wheat, they produce extra amounts of a protein called *zonulin*. The lining of the small intestine is basically a solid wall of cells that most materials can't pass through on their own. On the lining of the small intestine, zonulin waits for nutrients to come along. When important vitamins and minerals are present, zonulin tells the passageways in the intestinal wall to open so those nutrients can pass into the bloodstream. The blood then carries the nutrients to other parts of the body.

When some people eat wheat, they produce too much zonulin and the gates open too wide. All sorts of stuff gets into the bloodstream, some of which, like toxins, shouldn't be there. This increased permeability of the lining of the small intestine, or *leaky gut syndrome,* can cause lots of different health issues.

Discovering the Benefits of a Gluten-Free Lifestyle

Being gluten-free involves a lot more than just cutting gluten out of your diet. It affects every aspect of your life, from how you communicate and with whom, to how you handle ordering at restaurants, attending social functions, and dealing with emotional challenges.

I believe it's important to take control of your diet — or, if it's your kids who are gluten-free, help them gain and retain control. Going gluten-free also gives you an opportunity to reach out and help others who may be embarking upon the wonderful world of gluten free-dom, as well as a chance to discover more about nutrition and what you're actually putting into your body on a daily basis. If that sounds like a lot of work, relax. I guide you through it. And not only can you feel better, but you can also feel better about yourself!

You have lots of company. The gluten-free movement is sweeping the nation for plenty of reasons, but the one that stands out is that when people give up gluten, they often feel better. The following sections tell you what the gluten-free diet can do for your body — the benefits you can enjoy in addition to all the emotional perks of the lifestyle.

Eating isn't supposed to hurt

Food is fuel — it's supposed to give you energy and make you feel good, not make you hurt. But when you eat things that your body doesn't like for some reason, it has a sometimes not-so-subtle way of telling you to knock it off. Food that your body objects to can cause gas, bloating, diarrhea, constipation, and nausea — and even symptoms that don't seem to be associated with the gastrointestinal tract, such as headaches, fatigue, depression, joint pain, and respiratory distress.

Luckily, when you figure out which foods your body doesn't approve of, you can stop eating them, and then your body stops being so pouty. In fact, if you feed it right, your body can make you feel great in lots of different ways.

Making nutrition your mission: Head-to-toe health benefits

Twelfth-century physician Maimonides said, "Man should strive to have his intestines relaxed all the days of his life." No doubt! When your intestines aren't relaxed — or when they're downright edgy or uptight — they affect all your other body parts, too.

It's kind of like when you're in a really good mood and your best friend is grumpy — the situation can make you grumpy, too.

In a way, the body's reaction to gluten doesn't compute. For some people, eating gluten can cause headaches, fatigue, joint pain, depression, or infertility; at first, those types of symptoms may seem unrelated to something going on in your gut, much less something you eat — especially something as common in your diet as wheat.

But those problems — and about 250 others — are symptoms of celiac disease and gluten sensitivity. People with celiac disease or gluten sensitivity do sometimes have gastrointestinal symptoms, but more often the symptoms are *extraintestinal,* meaning they take place outside the intestinal tract.

If your body has problems with gluten, the gluten-free diet may help relieve lots of symptoms, such as

- ✔ Fatigue
- ✔ Gastrointestinal distress (gas, bloating, diarrhea, constipation, vomiting, heartburn, and acid reflux)
- ✔ Headaches (including migraines)
- ✔ Inability to concentrate
- ✔ Weight gain or weight loss
- ✔ Infertility
- ✔ Joint, bone, or muscle pain
- ✔ Depression
- ✔ Respiratory problems

The list's impressive, isn't it? The idea that eliminating one thing from your diet — gluten — could improve so many different conditions is almost hard to believe.

Yet it's true — and it really makes sense when you realize that if the food you're eating is toxic to your body, your body's going to scream in lots of different ways.

Note: In people with gluten intolerance, eating gluten may make the symptoms of some psychiatric conditions worse. Removing gluten from the diet can improve the behaviors of people with conditions such as autism, schizophrenia, and attention-deficit (hyperactivity) disorder.

Millions of people have wheat *allergies,* which are different from gluten sensitivity or celiac disease — and they, too, improve dramatically on a wheat-free/ gluten-free diet.

But beyond the obvious improvement you enjoy if you have an intolerance, other conditions and symptoms can improve on a wheat-free diet, such as PMS and menopausal symptoms. Eliminating wheat may even slow or reverse the signs of aging, reducing wrinkles and improving the tone and texture of skin.

Abstinence makes the gut grow stronger

When gluten is making you sick, what your symptoms are doesn't matter; even if your symptoms don't seem to be related to your gastrointestinal tract, nasty battles are going on inside your gut.

Hairlike structures called villi line your small intestine. The job of the villi is to increase the surface area of the small intestine so it can absorb more nutrients. Villi protrude (picture fingers sticking up) so that they have more surface area to absorb important nutrients.

For people who have gluten intolerance, the body sees gluten as a toxin and attacks the gluten molecule. In doing so, it also inadvertently attacks the villi, and those villi get blunted and shortened, sometimes to the extreme of becoming completely flat. This attack can reduce their ability to absorb nutrients — sometimes dramatically.

Blunted and flat villi can't absorb stuff so well, so those good-for-ya nutrients just slide right by and you don't get enough of the important vitamins, minerals, and other nutrients that are vital for good physical and emotional health. You may develop what's called *malabsorption* and become poorly nourished.

Don't worry! This story has a happy ending. Your villi are tenacious little things, and when you quit eating gluten, they begin to heal right away. Before you know it, your villi grow back and absorb nutrients again, and your health is fully restored. That's why I say abstinence makes the gut grow stronger.

By the way, lactase, which is the enzyme that breaks down the sugar lactose, is produced in the tip of the villi. When the villi get blunted, sometimes your ability to digest lactose decreases and you become lactose intolerant. When you quit eating gluten and the villi heal, you're usually able to tolerate dairy foods again.

Mastering the Meals

This book is about a lifestyle, not a diet. But no matter where that lifestyle takes you — eating in, eating out, attending social events, planning, shopping, preparing — being gluten-free all comes down to one thing: food.

Whether you're a kitchenphobe or a foodie, living a gluten-free lifestyle offers you an enormous selection

of foods and ingredients to choose from, as you discover in the next sections.

Planning and preparing

Putting together smart and healthful gluten-free meals
is a lot easier if you plan ahead. Walking through a
store, perusing restaurant menus, or (gasp!) sitting in
a bakery with a growling tummy isn't exactly condu-
cive to making good food choices.

 Give yourself a healthy advantage by planning
and even preparing meals in advance, especially
if your busy schedule has you eating away from
home frequently. If you know you'll be pressed
for time at breakfast or lunch, make your meals
the night before and bring healthful gluten-free
snacks in resealable plastic bags.

One of the coolest things about adopting a new
dietary lifestyle is exploring new and sometimes
unusual or unique foods. You may never have heard
of lots of gluten-free foods and ingredients, many of
which are not only delicious but also nutritional power-
houses. With the new perspective on food that the
gluten-free lifestyle can offer you, you may find yourself inspired to think outside the typical menu plan,
exploring unique and nutritious alternatives.

Shopping shrewdly

The healthiest way to enjoy a gluten-free lifestyle is to
eat things you can find at any grocery store or even a
farmers' market: meat, fish, seafood, fruits, and nonstarchy vegetables (see Chapter 4 for more tips on
shopping). If you want to add canned, processed, and
even junk foods to your shopping list, you can still do
most of your shopping at a regular grocery store, and
you can even buy generics.

If you hope to enjoy the delicious gluten-free specialty products that are available these days, you can find them in health food aisles or at health food stores or specialty shops. Or you can shop in your jammies on one of the many Internet sites specializing in gluten-free products (if you're using your library's Internet or an Internet café to shop online, I suggest you change out of your jammies).

Some people worry about the cost of the gluten-free lifestyle, but it doesn't have to be more expensive. I talk about eating gluten-free affordably in Chapter 4.

Considering your kitchen

For the most part, a gluten-free kitchen looks the same as any other kitchen — without the gluten, of course. You don't need to go out and buy special gadgets and tools, and you don't need two sets of pots, pans, utensils, or storage containers, either.

If you're sharing a kitchen with gluten, you need to be aware of some contamination issues so you don't inadvertently *glutenate* (contaminate with gluten) a perfectly good gluten-free meal. Keeping your crumbs to yourself isn't just a matter of hygiene — it can mean the difference between a meal you can eat and one you can't.

Some people find having separate areas in the pantry or cupboards for their gluten-free products to be helpful. This idea is especially good if you have gluten-free kids in the house because they can see that you always have lots of things on hand for them to eat, and they can quickly grab their favorite gluten-free goodies from their special area.

Cooking outside the recipe box

I believe if you give someone a recipe, you feed 'em for a meal. Show them how to make *anything* gluten-free, and you feed 'em for a lifetime. The point is, you can make anything gluten-free, and you're not constrained by recipes or the fact that you can't use regular flour or breadcrumbs. All you need is a little creativity and some basic guidelines for using gluten-free substitutions, which you can find in Chapter 5.

If you're a die-hard recipe fan, never fear — I give you ten tasty recipes in Chapter 7. Most of them are super simple to follow but leave your guests with the impression that you spent all day in the kitchen (and being thus indebted, they may volunteer to do the dishes).

Getting Excited about the Gluten-Free Lifestyle

Most people who embark on a gluten-free lifestyle are doing so because of health issues — and that means they have little or no choice in the matter. When people are forced to make changes in their routine, especially changes that affect what they can and can't eat, they're not always so quick to see the joy in the adjustments.

If you're a little gloomy about going from gluten-glommer to gluten-freebie, I understand. But prepare yourself to read about the scores of reasons to be excited about the gluten-free lifestyle.

"A" is for adapting your perspective on food

If you've been eating gluten (I believe that would make you a *glutenivore*) for a long time — say, for most of your life — then giving up foods as you know them may seem like a tough transition at first. Besides the obvious practical challenges of learning to ferret out gluten where it may be hidden, you have to deal with emotional, physical, social, and even financial challenges.

 You have to do only one thing to learn to love the gluten-free lifestyle: Adjust your perspective on food just a tinge. You really don't have to give up anything; you just have to make some modifications. The foods that used to be your favorites can still be your favorites if you want them to be, just in a slightly different form.

Or you may want to consider what may be a new and super-healthful approach for you: eating lean meats, fresh fruits, and nonstarchy vegetables. Again, you may have to tweak your perspective a bit before the diet feels natural to you, but it is, in fact, natural, nutritious, and naturally nutritious.

Savoring gluten-free flavors

People who are new to the concept of being gluten-free sometimes comment that the diet is boring. When I ask what they're eating, their cuisine routine usually centers on carrots and rice cakes. Who wouldn't be bored with that? That type of a diet is appalling, not appealing.

I *love* food. I love the flavor, the feeling of being full, and the nutritional value. Most of all, I love to explore foods I've never tried — as long as they're gluten-free, of course. I'd never encourage you to endure a diet of blandiose foods that could double as packing materials.

A healthful, gluten-free diet doesn't have to be boring or restrictive. You're not constrained to eating 32 individual portions of fruits and vegetables each day, like a rabbit nibbling nervously on carrots. If you enjoy bland foods, snaps for you. But if you think gluten-free has to be flavor-free, you're in for a pleasant surprise.

Getting out and about

You don't have to let the gluten-free lifestyle hold you back from doing anything you want to do. Well, okay, there are some things you can't do — like eat a pizza from the place around the corner or devour a stack of gluten-laden donuts. But as far as your activities and lifestyle are concerned, you can — and should — get out and about as you always have.

For the most part, ordering out isn't as easy as walking into a restaurant and asking for a gluten-free menu (a girl can dream). But eating at restaurants is definitely doable, and it's getting easier every day; you just need to start placing special orders, tuning in to contamination concerns, and asking questions.

Traveling is a breeze when you master eating at restaurants. Going to social events just requires a little advance planning, and holidays may barely faze you after you get the hang of going out in gluten-free style. Chapter 6 gives you more information on being gluten-free when you're out and about.

Raising kids to love the lifestyle

When my husband and I heard that our son Tyler would have to be gluten-free for the rest of his life, we were flooded with a bunch of emotions, most of which weren't very pleasant. At first, we felt burdened and overcome with grief and frustration, and we longed for the perfectly healthy little baby we thought we were entitled to. It was easy to focus on what we had lost and all that we'd have to change in our lives. But making adjustments didn't take long, and soon we'd learned not just to live the gluten-free lifestyle but to *love* it.

Most important, we wanted Tyler to love the lifestyle. After all, his diet, his life, and his future would be affected the most. Thankfully, Tyler does love the gluten-free lifestyle, and your kids can, too.

Lots of ideas are key in raising happy, healthy, gluten-free kids. Some of the highlights include giving them control of their diet from day one, always having yummy gluten-free treats on hand, reinforcing the benefits of the gluten-free lifestyle, and remembering that they're figuring out how to feel about the lifestyle from *you.* Promoting an optimistic outlook can instill a positive approach in them.

By the time your kids are teens, they should be in full control of their gluten-free diet. The most you can do is help them understand the diet and, just as important, the implications if they choose not to follow it. (Note that young adults away from home at college have a huge advantage these days because many colleges and universities now feature gluten-free menu options.)

Kids are flexible and resilient. Adopting a new lifestyle is usually harder for the parents than for the child.

Setting realistic expectations

Some people call me PollyDanna because they think I have an unrealistically optimistic view of the gluten-free lifestyle. It may be optimistic, but it's not unrealistic.

Setting reasonable expectations for what life will be like after you adopt a gluten-free lifestyle is important because you *will* encounter challenges and you need to be prepared to handle them well. Friends, family, and loved ones may not understand or accommodate your diet when you hope or expect they will. You may find social events to be overwhelming at first, or you may get confused or frustrated and feel like giving up on the diet. I assure you that you can overcome these trials and emerge stronger for them.

This book is the resource you need — wade your way through it and dog-ear the pages you want to come back to when you need some reminders for how to deal with difficult issues. And above all, keep an optimistic but realistic approach. If you do, you'll encounter fewer obstacles along the way.

Arming yourself with good information

The good news is that because the gluten-free diet is exploding in popularity, you can find lots of information about it. The bad news is that not all of that information is accurate.

Be leery of what you hear and read regarding all things gluten-free, and check the reliability of the source on everything. If you find conflicting information — and you will — dig deeper until you find out which source is right. Always keep a skeptical eye out for the good, the bad, and the completely ludicrous.

Chapter 2

Who's Going Gluten-Free and Why

. . . .

In This Chapter

▶ Looking at allergies, sensitivities, and disease

▶ Reviewing symptoms

▶ Undergoing the testing process

▶ Exploring the dangers of not going gluten-free

▶ Starting the healing process immediately

. . . .

So you've given up — or are considering giving up — gluten. You're definitely not alone. Millions of people are going gluten-free for a variety of reasons, and most of these individuals are seeing dramatic improvements in their health. The bottom line is that gluten doesn't sit well with a lot of people. That's because many (some even say *most*) people have some form of gluten sensitivity.

This chapter explains what gluten sensitivity is, how gluten can affect your body, and which tests can help you decide whether you need to go gluten-free.

Shedding Light on the Gluten-Sensitivity Spectrum

If you're like most people considering giving up gluten, you're doing so for one of the following reasons:

- ✔ A medical professional told you that you have to and that your health will improve if you do.

- ✔ You haven't been to any doctors, but you suspect you'll feel better on a gluten-free diet.

- ✔ You or your child has behavioral issues, and you believe a gluten-free diet will help.

Which group you fall into doesn't matter — you're probably right on all counts. Chances are, though, you didn't even consider giving up gluten until you suspected you had gluten sensitivity.

Gluten sensitivity is a physical sensitivity to gluten — hence the clever name. It's not easy to define because these sensitivities come in a variety of forms. Think of gluten sensitivities as falling somewhere on a spectrum, ranging from allergy to disease (see Figure 2-1). Don't let the word *spectrum* fool you, though. It's not a case of going from less severe to more severe; the types of sensitivities are just different. The next sections break down the parts of the spectrum.

At one end: Allergies

Technically, there's no such thing as an allergy to gluten, but a person can have allergies to foods or ingredients that contain gluten: wheat, rye, and barley. In fact, wheat is one of the most common allergens, affecting millions of people.

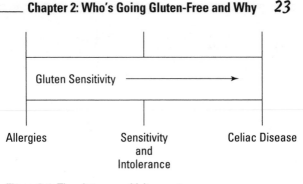

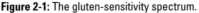

Figure 2-1: The gluten-sensitivity spectrum.

These allergies are just like other typical food allergies — the same as an allergy to strawberries or shellfish, for example. They're all responses to a food allergen, and the reaction that someone has to those foods varies from person to person and from one food to another.

Allergic symptoms can be respiratory, causing coughing, nasal congestion, sneezing, throat tightness, and even asthma.

Acute allergic reactions to food usually start in the mouth, with tingling, itching, a metallic taste, and swelling of the tongue and throat. Sometimes symptoms crop up farther down the intestinal tract, causing abdominal pain, muscle spasms, vomiting, and diarrhea.

Any severe and acute allergic reaction also has the potential to be life threatening, causing anaphylaxis. *Anaphylaxis* — or *anaphylactic shock* — affects different organs, and symptoms can include a tingling sensation, swelling in the mouth or throat, and a metallic taste. Other symptoms can include a feeling of agitation, hives, breathing problems, a drop in blood pressure, and fainting. Anaphylaxis can sometimes be fatal unless the person having the allergic reaction receives an epinephrine (adrenaline) injection.

Somewhere in the middle: Gluten sensitivity and intolerance

Moving across the spectrum of gluten sensitivity, you go from allergies into an ambiguous area that a lot of people call sensitivity or intolerance. Often used interchangeably, the terms *sensitivity* and *intolerance* basically mean that your body doesn't react well to a particular food and you should avoid it. Notice that I said *should,* not *must.*

What *is* clear is that people who fall into this area have a response to gluten that's very similar to a celiac response (which I talk about in the later "Identifying Symptoms of Gluten Sensitivity and Celiac Disease" section). So do they have celiac disease? Maybe. Here's where things get fuzzy:

- ✔ Some people who are diagnosed with gluten sensitivity actually have celiac disease, but their testing was done improperly or was insufficient to yield conclusive results.

- ✔ Other people may not have celiac disease — yet — but if they continue to eat gluten, they may develop it. (A condition in its early stages like this is sometimes referred to as *subclinical celiac disease.*)

- ✔ Still other people may not have celiac disease and may never get it. But they do have a sensitivity to gluten, and their health improves on a gluten-free diet.

Symptoms of gluten sensitivity are usually the same as those of celiac disease, and as with celiac disease, they usually go away on a gluten-free diet.

Testing can help clarify whether you have celiac disease or gluten sensitivity. If you test positive for celiac disease, then that's what you have. If you're negative for celiac disease yet your symptoms go away on a gluten-free diet, you probably have some form of gluten sensitivity.

To further complicate the issue, you may have gotten a *false* negative test result for celiac disease. This just means that your tests say you don't have celiac disease, but they're wrong. I talk more about this situation in the later "Getting Tested for Gluten Sensitivity and Celiac Disease" section).

Sadly, because protocol for defining and diagnosing gluten sensitivity isn't well established or practiced, patients are often told to ignore "inconclusive" or confusing test results and simply go back to eating their bagels and pizza. Sometimes this conclusion and "advice" can have serious and long-term harmful consequences for a patient's health.

Crossing the line: Celiac disease

Somewhere along the way on the gluten-sensitivity spectrum, the ambiguous sensitivity is no longer ambiguous: You have celiac disease. Unlike gluten sensitivity, celiac disease is well-defined.

Celiac disease is a common (yet often misdiagnosed) genetic intolerance to gluten. Triggered by eating gluten, the immune system responds by attacking the gluten molecule. In doing so, it also attacks your body cells (this is called an *autoimmune response*). The disease can develop at any age and in people of any ethnicity. It results in damage to the small intestine, which can cause poor absorption of nutrients. ***Note:*** Although the damage occurs in the gastrointestinal tract, not all symptoms are gastrointestinal in nature; in fact, symptoms are vast and varied, and they sometimes come and go, which makes diagnosis difficult.

Autism and behavioral disorders

Another type of gluten sensitivity is related to autism and other disorders on the autistic spectrum. A lot of the details about the "hows" and "whys" are still being ironed out, but noteworthy here is the fact that the gluten-free diet seems to have some role in improving these behavioral disorders.

Identifying Symptoms of Gluten Sensitivity and Celiac Disease

Many symptoms of celiac disease are also symptoms of gluten sensitivity, and they affect multiple parts of the body. That's because celiac disease is *multisystemic;* although the actual damage is occurring in the gastrointestinal tract — specifically, in the small intestine — the symptoms manifest in many different ways, in all different body parts.

Gluten sensitivity and celiac disease have hundreds of symptoms, so I can't list them all. The following sections give some of the more common symptoms, starting with the ones that are gastrointestinal in nature.

Getting a grip on gastrointestinal symptoms

Most people think the most common symptoms of celiac disease are gastrointestinal in nature — diarrhea, constipation, gas, bloating, reflux, and even vomiting. These are some of the "classic" — though not the most common — symptoms of celiac disease. Most people with celiac disease don't have gastrointestinal symptoms (even though damage is being done to their gastrointestinal tract). The "classic" gastrointestinal symptoms people get include the following:

- Abdominal pain and distension
- Acid reflux
- Bloating
- Constipation
- Diarrhea
- Gas and flatulence
- Greasy, foul-smelling, floating stools
- Nausea
- Vomiting
- Weight loss or weight gain

Identifying nongastrointestinal symptoms

Interestingly, although gluten sensitivity and celiac disease affect the gut, most people's symptoms aren't gastrointestinal in nature. People more commonly have what are called *extraintestinal symptoms;* the list of these is extensive, more than 250. The following is only a partial listing:

- Fatigue and weakness (due to iron-deficiency anemia)
- Vitamin and/or mineral deficiencies
- Headaches (including migraines)
- Joint/bone pain
- Depression, irritability, listlessness, and mood disorders
- "Fuzzy brain" or an inability to concentrate

✔ Infertility

✔ Abnormal menstrual cycles

✔ Dental enamel deficiencies and irregularities

✔ Seizures

Celiac disease can also be associated with thyroid disease — usually hypothyroidism — and that itself can lead to dry skin.

Spotting symptoms in kids

Kids who have celiac disease tend to have the "classic" gastrointestinal symptoms of diarrhea or constipation, but there are certainly other symptoms to look for, including

✔ Inability to concentrate

✔ Irritability

✔ ADD/ADHD or autistic-type behaviors

✔ Failure to thrive (in infants and toddlers)

✔ Short stature or delayed growth

✔ Delayed onset of puberty

✔ Weak bones or bone pain

✔ Abdominal pain and distension

✔ Nosebleeds

Discovering misdiagnoses and the missed diagnoses

In Europe, the average time between the onset of symptoms and a diagnosis of celiac disease is six months. In the United States, if the diagnosis ever comes, it takes an average of 11 years after symptoms develop.

When no symptoms are a symptom

Some people have no noticeable symptoms whatsoever — these people are called *asymptomatic*. But even though they don't feel any symptoms, gluten is damaging their small intestine, which can result in nutritional deficiencies and associated conditions. These people have it tough, in terms of both diagnosis and treatment. They usually get diagnosed because they have a relative who has celiac disease and they're smart enough to know that means they should be tested, too. As for treatment, they need to be gluten-free in order to be healthy. But it's tough to stay motivated to give up some of your favorite foods when those foods don't seem to make you feel bad!

A *Reader's Digest* article titled "10 Diseases Doctors Miss" cited celiac disease as one of the top ten misdiagnosed diseases. For every person diagnosed with celiac disease, 140 go undiagnosed. And that doesn't even account for the population that has gluten sensitivity (not celiac disease) and may never know it.

As awareness of celiac disease and gluten sensitivity is increasing, diagnoses are on the rise, and people are discovering improved health on a gluten-free diet. However, underdiagnosis is still a big problem. Patients are often misdiagnosed with a variety of maladies before finding out that they really have celiac disease — something that's easily cured by diet. Common misdiagnoses include

- Irritable bowel syndrome (IBS) or spastic colon
- Chronic fatigue syndrome (CFS) or fibromyalgia
- Lupus (an autoimmune disease)
- Unexplained anemia

- ✔ Migraines or unexplained headaches
- ✔ Unexplained infertility
- ✔ Psychological issues (hypochondria, depression, anxiety, or neurosis)
- ✔ Inflammatory bowel disease (IBD), such as Crohn's disease and colitis
- ✔ Cancer
- ✔ Viral infections (viral gastroenteritis)

Why the diagnosis is missed

Gluten sensitivity and celiac disease are common and can cause severe problems if undiagnosed. Yet most people with gluten sensitivity or celiac disease go undiagnosed or misdiagnosed. Why are doctors missing the diagnosis of this common condition? Michelle Pietzak, MD, one of the foremost experts on celiac disease, offers some ideas:

- ✔ Physicians aren't exposed to it enough in medical school and residency training.
- ✔ Some doctors get "continuing medical information" from drug reps, journal articles, and conferences.
- ✔ Symptoms are vast and sometimes even absent.
- ✔ Physicians may think the patients are exaggerating or just plain "crazy."
- ✔ Physicians may be uncomfortable if they feel ignorant.
- ✔ Routine blood tests don't pick it up.
- ✔ Routine endoscopies and poorly done biopsies don't detect celiac disease.
- ✔ Cost-containment in the medical field may limit testing.

What's a shame about these misdiagnoses is that many patients who are diagnosed with these conditions are either told that nothing can be done or put on drug regimes that, by definition, have side effects. Both of these scenarios are unfortunate, especially considering that the real answer might lie simply in a dietary modification.

Getting Tested for Gluten Sensitivity and Celiac Disease

Testing for gluten sensitivity and celiac disease isn't an exact science — nor do "exact scientists" agree on protocol for some of the testing procedures available today. The sections that follow fill you in on the types of tests available, give you guidance on interpreting your test results, and help you figure out next steps if you test positive.

Surveying the different testing protocols

The most widely accepted testing protocol for celiac disease includes a blood test followed by an intestinal biopsy.

  ✔ **Blood tests:** Also called *serological tests,* blood tests look for five antibodies that the body produces when someone with a sensitivity or celiac disease eats gluten — tTG-IgA, EMA-IgA, AGA-IgA, AGA-IgG, and Total serum IgA. Any lab can draw the blood as long as you have an order from a health care practitioner who's allowed to order blood draws; the lab technicians can get the blood they need for all the necessary tests with a single blood draw. If any of the blood tests are positive, the results may indicate celiac disease or gluten sensitivity. Your doctor will probably want to do an intestinal biopsy to confirm the diagnosis.

✔ **Biopsies:** Biopsies are considered the gold standard for diagnosing celiac disease. When doctors do a biopsy, they do it by way of an endoscopy: They put a tube down your throat to the small intestine and then clip samples of the *villi,* hairlike structures on the lining of the small intestine. When people with celiac disease eat gluten, the body launches an attack and ends up turning on itself, blunting the villi. A biopsy determines how much blunting, if any, has occurred.

The endoscopy itself and the clipping of the villi aren't painful. However, a biopsy *is* an invasive procedure, so some risks are involved. Adults are usually sedated with drugs like Versed (midazolam) and Demerol (meperidine); children usually require a general anesthetic.

You have to be eating gluten for an extended length of time before blood or biopsy testing. If you don't eat gluten, or haven't eaten it for long enough, your body may not produce enough antibodies to show up on the blood tests, and the results will seem to show that you're "normal" — or "negative" for gluten sensitivity or celiac disease. Same goes for the biopsy — if you're not eating gluten, your small intestine will be healing or healed, and the biopsy will be negative for celiac disease.

Other testing options include the following:

✔ **Stool tests:** At least one lab does home stool-testing for gluten sensitivity, microscopic colitis, genetic susceptibility, and several other gastrointestinal conditions. Like the blood test, the stool test looks for the immune system's reactions to gluten by detecting the presence of certain antibodies. The lab sends you a convenient container; you just do your business in it and send it back by overnight mail. The most established lab doing this testing in the United States is EnteroLab.

✔ **Genetic tests:** These tests look to see whether a person has the genes associated with celiac disease and can be done by blood, stool, or a new saliva home test. Genetic testing is valuable for ruling out celiac disease because if your body doesn't produce either protein HLA-DQ2 or HLA-DQ8, there's a 99 percent chance you don't have celiac disease. The test isn't valuable for predicting who will get celiac disease, though, because lots of people have these genes and never develop the disease.

MyCeliacID (www.myceliacid.com) is a new saliva-based home-testing kit that does genetic testing for celiac disease. You order a kit online, spit in the tube, and send it back. Within a matter of days, you have your results. This is a highly specific test that looks for "risk stratification," meaning it can tell you not only whether you have celiac disease but also how likely you are to get it.

Many patients have told me that their doctor ordered a colonoscopy to test for celiac disease. A colonoscopy is not a test for celiac disease (it's the wrong end of the body). If your doctor orders a colonoscopy, it should only be to test for other conditions — if he or she says it's to test for celiac disease, ask more questions to make sure you're both understanding the testing procedures.

Interpreting your test results

Sometimes interpretation of your test results is straightforward; other times it's not even close.

For one thing, false negatives and, occasionally, false positives can occur. False negatives can arise from several factors, including the following:

- ✔ Testing is somewhat subjective, and not all labs do it well. Many lab technicians rarely, if ever, see celiac panels and don't always do them properly.

- ✔ Different pathologists read biopsies differently. Some, for instance, believe that mild blunting of the villi indicates celiac disease; others think celiac disease is a possible diagnosis only if the villi are completely blunted.

- ✔ Not eating enough gluten prior to testing can affect the amount of antibodies you produce.

- ✔ Testing that doesn't include all five blood tests may leave an antibody unnoticed.

 Celiac disease and gluten sensitivity can be triggered at any age, so just because you tested negative once doesn't mean you're "out of the woods" forever. Lots of people say, "I was tested for celiac disease, and I don't have it." Wrong assumption. You may have tested negative once upon a time, but the disease may have been triggered since then.

I realize there are endless iterations of the chart I've put together for you in Table 2-1, but I couldn't possibly include all the various combinations. So for the most part, tests can be interpreted like this (note that this chart assumes you're not IgA deficient, so IgA-based tests are conclusive).

Table 2-1	Interpreting Your Test Results
Test Result	**Likely Diagnosis**
Positive EMA, tTG, or biopsy (regardless of AGA-IgA and IgG results)	Celiac disease likely. Step away from the pizza.
Negative EMA, tTG, and biopsy Positive AGA-IgA and IgG	Most likely not celiac disease, but could be gluten sensitivity. Forget the donuts.
Positive AGA-IgG All other tests negative	Could be gluten sensitivity or another leaky gut syndrome.
All tests negative	Seemingly no problem with gluten. Enjoy all the pizza and donuts you like. (But don't blame me when your pants don't fit!)

Some people test negative on some or all of the tests, yet they find that they don't feel right when they eat gluten. Perhaps you got false negatives — or maybe gluten just doesn't sit right with you. Bottom line: If it makes you feel bad, don't eat it!

Figuring out what to do if you test positive

If you've tested positive, your next step depends on what you tested positive for. It also depends on whether you had the complete testing panels done. If you're positive for

✔ **Gluten sensitivity:** You may be able to get away with eating gluten from time to time. But before you start diving into your favorite pizza, you may want to make sure you're really negative for celiac disease because sometimes people are told they're gluten sensitive when, in fact, they have celiac disease. If that's the case and you go back to eating gluten, you could be doing some hefty damage every time you indulge. Ask yourself and your doctor these questions:

- Were all the tests for celiac disease done?

- Were the results "iffy" or "inconclusive," or were they definitive?

- If a child is being tested, is the child old enough (over the age of 2) to show an antibody response?

If you aren't sure you can trust your test results, you may want to be tested again somewhere down the line.

✔ **Celiac disease:** If you've been diagnosed with celiac disease, you're in luck because you already know the key to your better health: a gluten-free lifestyle. Going gluten-free right away is important. You may make mistakes at first, and that's okay. Learn from them and move on.

Keep in mind that celiac disease is a genetic condition. If you've been diagnosed, your family members need to be tested, too.

✔ **Wheat allergies:** Although the conditions are different, you could have an allergy *and* a gluten sensitivity or celiac disease. So if you're diagnosed with wheat allergies, make sure you're also tested for the more global conditions of gluten sensitivity and celiac disease so you know just what dietary guidelines you need to follow.

If you're not positive for those but have only a wheat allergy, you need to avoid wheat but can still eat rye and barley. And if you suspect you may have an anaphylactic response, consider carrying an EpiPen (or another brand of epinephrine shot that allows you to inject yourself) in case you accidentally eat wheat.

Considering the Risks If You Don't Give Up Gluten

Invariably, at least four groups of people decide they're going to continue to eat gluten even if they have problems with it:

- ✔ People who think the diet is too restrictive, so they're not going to bother trying

- ✔ People who don't feel symptoms or were never properly diagnosed and figure that cheating from time to time is okay

- ✔ People who feel symptoms but figure the discomfort is worth the chance to enjoy a few beers (or any other glutenous favorite) from time to time

- ✔ Relatives who refuse to hear anything about gluten

If you fall into one of these categories and refuse to give up gluten even though you have or suspect you may have gluten sensitivity or celiac disease, there's not much anyone can do. But before you finish your donut, at least read the next two sections, which cover the conditions associated with celiac disease — and the serious complications that can arise if you continue to eat gluten.

Looking at associated conditions

Certain conditions are associated with celiac disease, meaning someone who has one is more likely to have the other. It's not always clear which one developed first (except, for instance, Down syndrome, which people are born with), but if you don't give up gluten, your chances of developing some of these conditions may increase.

Also, if you have one of these conditions but haven't been tested for gluten sensitivity or celiac disease, you should be tested because the two go hand in hand; the fact that you have one of these diseases is a red flag that you may also have gluten sensitivity or celiac disease.

- ✔ **Autoimmune diseases:** Several autoimmune diseases are associated with celiac disease, including Addison's disease, Crohn's disease, insulin-dependent diabetes mellitus (Type 1), Sjögren's syndrome, and thyroid disease (specifically Graves' disease and Hashimoto's disease).

- ✔ **Mood disorders:** Some of the mood disorders associated with gluten sensitivity and celiac disease include attention-deficit (hyperactive) disorder (ADD/ADHD), autism, depression and bipolar disease, and schizophrenia.

- ✔ **Nutritional deficiencies:** Because gluten sensitivity and celiac disease affect the small intestine, nutritional deficiencies are associated. In addition to specific vitamin and mineral deficiencies, people may have anemia; osteoporosis, osteopenia, or osteomalacia; or the myriad conditions that arise due to nutritional deficiencies.

✔ **Neurological conditions:** Some neurological conditions are associated with gluten sensitivity and celiac disease, including epilepsy and cerebral calcifications; brain and spinal cord defects; and neurological problems such as ataxia, neuropathy, tingling, seizures, and optic myopathy.

✔ **Other conditions:** Several other conditions are commonly associated with celiac disease, including cancer, Down syndrome, internal hemorrhaging, organ disorders (of the gallbladder, liver, spleen, or pancreas), tooth enamel defects, and cystic fibrosis.

Type 1 diabetes and celiac disease often go hand in hand. About 6 percent of people with Type 1 diabetes have celiac disease, but many don't know it. People with celiac disease and Type 1 diabetes often find managing blood-sugar levels is much easier on the gluten-free diet.

The earlier in life you go on a gluten-free diet, the lower your risk of developing associated conditions. And sometimes symptoms of other autoimmune diseases, like multiple sclerosis, improve on a gluten-free diet.

Living with compromised health

You may feel perfectly healthy. You may be *asymptomatic* (have no apparent symptoms) or have mild symptoms that you barely notice. But if you have gluten sensitivity or celiac disease and you continue to eat gluten, you're doubtlessly compromising your health because your body is being robbed of important nutrients that it needs to function properly and stay strong.

Many people say that they didn't realize how bad they felt until they went gluten-free. Then they enjoy such improved and even optimal health that they realize that eating gluten compromised their health, and they didn't even know it.

Healing Begins on Day One

One of the coolest things about going gluten-free when you have gluten sensitivity or celiac disease is that you start healing the minute you start on the diet.

Most people begin feeling better immediately, some take months to improve, and some feel better initially but then take a nosedive a few months into the diet. All of these are normal responses to your body's healing process, and in the long run, you can look forward to improved health in ways you may not have even expected.

 Although most, if not all, of the intestinal damage caused by gluten is reversible, some of the prolonged malnutrition and malabsorption issues, such as short stature and weakened bones, may have long-lasting, if not permanent, effects. That's one of the reasons why catching gluten sensitivity or celiac disease early is important — so you can start skipping down the road to recovery.

Chapter 3

Grasping the Diet's Ground Rules

*T*he gluten-free diet seems like it should be so easy: Gluten is in wheat, rye, and barley — so just avoid those foods, right? If the diet were that simple, I'd be signing off with "The End" or "Love, Danna" right about now, and the book would be finished. No, the diet's not quite that straightforward thanks to additives, flavorings, derivatives, fillers, binders, and other fancy terms that are really just euphemisms for "stuff that may have gluten in it." But the good news is that the list of foods you can eat is a lot longer than the list of foods you can't.

Whether you're a one or a ten on the I'm-overwhelmed-by-this-diet scale, this chapter is key because it establishes basic gluten-free guidelines. I outline what is and isn't gluten-free and why you sometimes have to question a product. I introduce you to gluten-free alternatives that you may never have heard of. I also talk about nonfood items that you may or may not need to be concerned about, such as dental products, alcoholic beverages, medications, and external products like lotions and shampoos.

When in Doubt, Leave It Out

I can say unequivocally that at some point, you're going to wonder whether a product is gluten-free. You may be at a restaurant or party and have no idea what's in the food. The labeling may not be clear, there may not be any labels in sight, or you may not know half the words on the label. Don't assume that because you don't *know* that something's *not* okay that it's safe for you to eat. If you need a reminder of what you're doing to your body when you eat gluten, take a look at Chapter 2, which talks about associated conditions and serious complications that can develop if you have gluten sensitivity or celiac disease and eat gluten.

Even if your symptoms are mild or absent, the damage gluten causes — even small amounts of gluten — can be severe. You're a lot better off being safe instead of sorry, so follow this common-sense commandment: When in doubt, leave it out.

Defining Gluten So You Can Avoid It

You have to know what gluten is — and not just so you can be the life of the party, sparking tantalizing conversations that begin with audacious lines like, "So, which do you find harder to avoid? Gliadin, hordein, or secalin?" No, you need to know about gluten so you can avoid it. The definition of gluten is so convoluted that it's hard to offer a technically correct one at this point, but I'll give it a whirl.

Gluten is what scientists call a storage protein, what bakers call the dough-forming elastic ingredient in wheat, and what some newbies to the gluten-free diet pine away for. It's a group of proteins that technically comes from wheat and only wheat.

At some point in our not-so-distant history, someone made the association between wheat (specifically, gluten) and celiac disease. People widely accepted that gluten makes celiacs sick, which is true. Soon physicians realized that barley and rye make celiacs sick, too, and people started saying, "Celiacs can't eat gluten. They can't eat wheat, barley, and rye, either; therefore, wheat, barley, and rye all have gluten." Right? Kind of, but not really. One of the types of proteins in gluten is also in barley and rye.

The "wheat, barley, and rye (and maybe oats) all have gluten" idea stuck, and even though it isn't technically correct, it *is* widely accepted today. For the purposes of this book, I stick with it, too.

Wheat-free doesn't mean *gluten-free*. Something can be wheat-free and still have, for instance, malt (derived from barley), so then it's not gluten-free.

Recognizing Gluten-Free Foods at a Glance

Keep in mind that you have to become familiar with lots of ingredients when you're diving into the gluten-free diet. The reason the gluten-free diet can seem

cumbersome at first is that "derivatives" of gluten-
containing grains may contain gluten. Then, of course,
processed foods — which contain seasonings, additives, and flavorings — can contain ingredients that
raise questions, too.

But breaking foods down into those that usually have
gluten and those that don't isn't too tough, which is
why I've done that for you in the following sections.
Keep in mind, though, that these lists vary and are
only to get you started. You can find up-to-date lists
of foods that are safe, forbidden, and questionable at
www.celiac.com.

Forbidden grains

I'm not starting with the forbidden grains to be
negative — I'm starting with them because the list
is a lot shorter than the list of grains you can eat (see
the later related section). You need to avoid these
grains on a gluten-free diet:

- Barley

- Oats (because of contamination issues)

- Rye

- Triticale (a hybrid of wheat and rye)

- Wheat

You need to avoid (or at least question) anything with the word *wheat* in it. This includes
hydrolyzed wheat protein, wheat starch, wheat
germ, and so on. Wheat grass, however, like all
grasses, is gluten-free, but you still need to
make sure you're not dealing with contamination from sprouts (see the later "Grasses,
sprouted grains, berries, and bran" sidebar for
more on this topic).

Here are a few additional details worth keeping in mind:

- ✔ Wheat starch is actually wheat that has had the gluten washed out. In some countries, a special type of wheat starch called Codex Alimentarius wheat starch is allowed on the gluten-free diet — but it's not allowed in North America because some people question whether the washing process completely removes all residual gluten.

- ✔ Triticale is a made-up grain — a hybrid of wheat and rye. Inventors developed it to combine the productivity of wheat with the ruggedness of rye. Relatively speaking, it's fairly nutritious for people who can eat gluten.

- ✔ Wheat has several names and varieties. Beware of aliases like *flour, bulgur, semolina, spelt, frumento, durum* (also spelled *duram*), *kamut, graham, einkorn, farina, couscous, seitan, matzoh, matzah, matzo,* and *cake flour.* Often marketed as a "wheat alternative," spelt is as much of a wheat alternative as I am a human alternative. It's not even remotely gluten-free. Einkorn and emmer are sometimes touted as being safe, but they too contain harmful prolamins and must be avoided on a gluten-free diet.

- ✔ Wheat just isn't what it used to be. In fact, in an effort to bring down the cost of commercial baked goods and make wheat slightly more nutritious for the countries the United States ships to, ambitious farmers are actually finding ways to hybridize wheat to make it have more gluten than ever.

- ✔ Derivatives of gluten-containing grains aren't allowed on the gluten-free diet, either. You can find a complete listing at www.celiac.com, but the most common derivative that you have to avoid is malt, which usually comes from barley. Avoid malt, malt flavoring, and malt vinegar. *Note:* If malt is derived from another source, such as corn, that fact usually appears on the label; if it's not specified, though, don't eat it.

Grains and starches you can safely eat

You have lots of choices for gluten-free grains and starches. Even if you're an old pro who's been gluten-free for years, I'm guessing some of these may be new to you:

- ✔ Amaranth
- ✔ Arrowroot
- ✔ Beans
- ✔ Buckwheat/groats/kasha
- ✔ Chickpeas (garbanzo beans, besan, cici, chana, or gram — not to be confused with graham, which does have gluten)
- ✔ Corn
- ✔ Garfava
- ✔ Job's Tears
- ✔ Mesquite (pinole)
- ✔ Millet
- ✔ Montina (Indian ricegrass)
- ✔ Oats (but they may be contaminated with wheat and other grains)
- ✔ Potato
- ✔ Quinoa (hie)
- ✔ Ragi

- ✔ Rice
- ✔ Sorghum
- ✔ Soy
- ✔ Tapioca (gari, cassava, casaba, manioc, yucca)
- ✔ Taro root
- ✔ Teff

Glutinous rice doesn't contain gluten! Manufacturers make glutinous rice, also called *sweet rice* or *mochi,* by grinding high-starch, short-grain rice. Glutinous rice thickens sauces and desserts in Asian cooking and is often the rice used in sushi.

Grasses, sprouted grains, berries, and bran

Grasses such as wheat grass and barley grass, frequently sold in health food stores and at juice bars, are gluten-free. The grass hasn't yet formed the gluten-containing proteins that cause problems in people with gluten sensitivity and celiac disease. When you can watch someone cut the grass so you know it's fresh and hasn't sprouted yet, you're safe. Be careful, though, of grasses that are an ingredient in a product. These grasses could be contaminated with seeds, and because you don't know for sure, you could risk getting gluten.

You should avoid sprouted grains because you don't know where in the sprouting process the grain is. Eating the sprouts could be okay, but it may not be. Berries are the seed kernels and are definitely not safe. The jury's still out on bran, so until food scientists do more research, remember the common-sense commandment I refer to in this chapter: *When in doubt, leave it out.*

So you want to sow your oats . . .

There's no clear-cut (or steel-cut) answer on oats — yet. Most people agree that, in and of themselves, oats are gluten-free (although at least one study showed otherwise), but when processed commercially, they can become contaminated during the manufacturing process.

Some people argue that the risk of contamination is extremely low — you still need to assess whether you're willing to take that risk. Some companies certify that their oats are gluten-free. They're grown in dedicated fields and are harvested and processed with dedicated gluten-free machinery. Those oats are your best bet.

Bottom line: If you can find pure, uncontaminated oats, they may not present a problem.

You may run across different names or forms of corn that are gluten-free in addition to plain ol' corn. They include grits, hominy, masa, masa harina, harinilla (blue corn), atole, maize, polenta, corn gluten, and, of course, cornstarch, corn flour, corn bran, and cornmeal.

Gums, such as xanthan and guar, contain no gluten. People use them frequently in gluten-free baked goods because gums help give the spongy, elastic texture that gluten-containing flours usually provide. *Note:* For some people, gums — especially guar gum — may have a laxative effect.

Other foods that are usually gluten-free

In general, the following foods are usually gluten-free (note that this list refers to plain, unseasoned foods without additives and processed products):

- ✔ Beans
- ✔ Dairy products
- ✔ Eggs
- ✔ Fish
- ✔ Fruit
- ✔ Legumes
- ✔ Meat
- ✔ Nuts
- ✔ Poultry
- ✔ Seafood
- ✔ Vegetables

You can buy specialty products such as cookies, cakes, brownies, breads, crackers, and pretzels that have been made with gluten-free ingredients. I talk more about those products and where to buy them in Chapter 4, which covers shopping.

Foods that usually contain gluten

Companies offer special gluten-free varieties of some foods, and those gluten-free varieties obviously don't have gluten in them. But unless you're buying specialty products, you can assume that the following foods contain gluten:

- ✔ Beer
- ✔ Bread, breadcrumbs, biscuits
- ✔ Cereal
- ✔ Communion wafers
- ✔ Cookies, cakes, cupcakes, donuts, muffins, pastries, pie crusts, brownies, and other baked goods
- ✔ Cornbread

✔ Crackers

✔ Croutons

✔ Gravies, sauces, and roux

✔ Imitation seafood (for example, imitation crab)

✔ Licorice

✔ Marinades (such as teriyaki)

✔ Pasta

✔ Pizza crust

✔ Pretzels

✔ Soy sauce

✔ Stuffing

Exploring Alternative Grains

When it comes to grains beyond corn, wheat, and rice, most people don't know barley from bulgur. But there's a great big world of grains out there to be explored, many of which are gluten-free, delicious, and loaded with nutritional value.

Don't eat the wheat meat

Seitan, pronounced say-*tahn,* is a chewy food made from gluten that resembles meat in texture. Also called *wheat meat,* seitan is made by making dough out of wheat flour and water, kneading it to develop the gluten, and rinsing away the starch and bran, leaving only the gluten. It's then simmered in water or vegetable broth that has been seasoned with soy sauce, resulting in a chewy, firm, meatlike food . . . food that's not only *loaded* with gluten but actually *is* gluten.

They're called *alternative grains,* yet many aren't grains at all. Instead, they're grasses, seeds, or flowers. People also call them *superfoods* because they're foods that are *super* nutritious. Take a look at some of the alternative grains I describe in the next sections and discover an entirely new world of gluten-free superfoods.

Note: For years, rumors have spread that some of these alternative grains aren't safe for people with gluten sensitivity or celiac disease. These foods are, in fact, gluten-free. Some people may have had reactions to these grains (as they would to corn, soy, or other allergens or foods to which they may have a sensitivity), but it's not a gluten reaction. But regardless of whether a food contains gluten, if it makes you sick, don't eat it!

Amaranth

Loaded with fiber, iron, calcium, and other vitamins and minerals, amaranth is also high in the amino acids lysine, methionine, and cysteine, and it's an excellent source of protein. A small beadlike grain, amaranth is not only nutritious but also delicious, with a pleasant peppery and hearty nutty flavor.

Amaranth isn't a true cereal grain at all; it's actually a relative of the pigweeds and ornamental flowers called *cockscomb.* People grow it not only for its seed but also for its leaves, which you can cook and eat as greens. Amaranth can be milled or toasted, which gives it extra flavor. You can even pop some varieties like popcorn, boil and eat them like cereal, or use them in soups and granolas or as a side dish.

You should always cook amaranth before eating it because, like some other edible seeds, it contains compounds that can inhibit the proper absorption of certain nutrients.

Arrowroot

Once revered by the ancient Mayans and other inhabitants of Central America as an antidote to poison arrows, arrowroot is now used as an herb and thought to soothe the stomach and have antidiarrheal effects. People use it in cooking as a thickener for soups, sauces, and confections.

An easily digested and nutritious starch, arrowroot is a fine white powder with a look and texture similar to that of cornstarch. The translucent paste has no flavor and sets to an almost clear gel. You can use arrowroot in gluten-free cooking or as a thickening agent to replace cornstarch, although it thickens at a lower temperature than either cornstarch or wheat, and its consistency doesn't hold as long after cooking. The superfine grains are easy to digest, making arrowroot a perfect "invalid" food. (In fact, arrowroot biscuits are one of the first solid foods babies can safely eat, but beware — manufacturers usually add wheat flour to arrowroot biscuits, so they're not gluten-free.)

Buckwheat (soba)

The fact that buckwheat is gluten-free often confuses people; after all, buckwheat has the word *wheat* right in the name. But buckwheat isn't even related to wheat; in fact, it's not even a true cereal grain. It's a fruit, a distant cousin of garden-variety rhubarb. The buckwheat seed has a three-cornered shell that contains a pale kernel known as a *groat.* In one form or another, groats have been around since the tenth century B.C.

High in lysine, which is an amino acid lacking in many traditional grains, buckwheat contains several other amino acids — in fact, this grain has a high proportion of all eight essential amino acids, which the human body doesn't make but still needs to keep functioning. In that way, buckwheat is closer to being a complete protein than many other plant sources. It's also high in many of the B vitamins, as well as the minerals phosphorus, magnesium, iron, copper, manganese, and zinc. And buckwheat is a good source of linoleic acid, an essential fatty acid.

Whole white buckwheat is naturally dried and has a delicate flavor that makes it a good stand-in for rice or pasta. When the hulled buckwheat kernels are roasted, they're called *kasha,* which has a deep tan color, a nutty flavor, and a slightly scorched smell. Cooks often use buckwheat in pancakes, biscuits, and muffins — but be aware that manufacturers often combine buckwheat with wheat in those products, so you have to read the labels carefully before buying buckwheat products. In Japan, people often make buckwheat into *soba,* or noodles, which sometimes — but not always — have wheat flour as well.

Mesquite (pinole)

Most people know of mesquite as an on-the-grill flavoring that makes foods taste smoky and sweet. But mesquite has been a staple for Native Americans for thousands of years. Its sweet, fragrant flowers make a honeylike substance, and the pod produces a ground meal called *pinole.* Mesquite flour is helpful in controlling blood sugar levels. Furthermore, soluble fibers in the seeds and pods slow the absorption of nutrients, which also helps in managing blood sugar.

The sweet pods and seeds are a good source of fiber, calcium, manganese, iron, and zinc. They're also high in protein, and they contain the amino acid lysine, which isn't present in many traditional grains. Not only does mesquite flour stabilize blood sugar but it also tastes great, with a sweet, slightly nutty flavor that bears a hint of molasses.

Mixes that combine mesquite with other gluten-free flours are now available, making creating gluten-free goodies with this unique flour a snap.

Millet

Not a grain at all, millet is actually a grass with small, round, ivory and yellow kernels that swell when you cook them. Millet supplies more servings per pound than any other grain.

Millet is packed with vitamins, minerals, and other nutrients. High in iron, magnesium, phosphorus, and potassium, it's also loaded with fiber and protein, as well as the B-complex vitamins, including niacin, thiamin, and riboflavin. Millet is more alkaline (meaning it has a higher pH) than many traditional grains and is very easy to digest.

Montina (Indian ricegrass)

Montina is actually Amazing Grains's trademarked name for Indian ricegrass. Indian ricegrass was a dietary staple of Native American cultures from the Southwest United States to Canada more than 7,000 years ago. Extremely hearty, Indian ricegrass was a good substitute during years when maize crops failed or game was in short supply. It has a bold flavor and is loaded with fiber and protein.

Quinoa (hie)

Quinoa (pronounced *keen*-wa) — and also called *hie* (pronounced *he*-uh) — is yet another of the grains that isn't really a grain; it's actually a fruit and a relative of the common weed lambsquarter. The National Academy of Science describes quinoa as "the most nearly perfect source of protein from the vegetable kingdom."

Like other superfoods and alternative grains, quinoa is packed with lysine and other amino acids that make it a complete protein. It's also high in phosphorus, calcium, iron, vitamin E, and assorted B vitamins, as well as fiber. Quinoa is usually pale yellow in color, but it also comes in pink, orange, red, purple, and black.

Because the uncooked grains are coated with *saponins* — sticky, bitter-tasting stuff that acts as a natural insect repellent — you should rinse quinoa thoroughly before cooking.

Sorghum (milo, jowar, jowari, cholam)

Sorghum is another of the oldest-known grains (that isn't a true cereal grain), and it has been a major source of nutrition in Africa and India for centuries. Now also grown in the United States, sorghum is generating excitement as a gluten-free insoluble fiber and is probably best known for the syrup that comes from one of its varieties.

Because sorghum's protein and starch are more slowly digested than that of other cereals, it may be beneficial to diabetics (and healthful for anyone). It's high in iron, calcium, and potassium, and doctors actually used to prescribe it as a supplement for people low in these nutrients.

Sorghum fans boast of its bland flavor and light color, which don't alter the taste or look of foods when you use sorghum in place of wheat flour. Many cooks suggest combining sorghum with soybean flour. Sorghum is also fermented and used in alcoholic beverages.

Teff (tef)

Although tiny, teff is a nutritional powerhouse. It's the smallest of the grains that aren't true cereal grains. A staple grain in Ethiopia for nearly 5,000 years, teff packs a protein content of nearly 12 percent and is five times richer in calcium, iron, and potassium than any other grain. Teff, which has a sweet, nutty flavor, grows in many different varieties and colors, but the most common are ivory, brown, and reddish-tan varieties.

You can cook the whole grain and serve it with sliced fruit or as a breakfast cereal with butter and brown sugar on top. Or you can add teff flour to baked goods to add a unique flavor and beef up the nutritional value.

If you've heard of teff, it's probably in reference to *injera,* a traditional fermented bread with a spongy texture and yeasty taste. Treated as an edible utensil, injera is used to soak up juices and soups, and even to grab meat and eat it. Beware, though; traditional injera has wheat flour added to it.

Checking Up on Questionable Ingredients

The gluten-free diet gets a little trickier when you don't know that a food is almost always gluten-free or gluten-loaded. In the sections that follow, I go over what items you need to question and I discuss some of the foods people used to question but now know are gluten-free.

The facts on flavorings

Flavorings have been considered a questionable ingredient on the gluten-free diet for years. But according to Shelley Case, one of the leading authorities on the gluten-free diet, there's little or no need to question flavorings anymore. She points out that gluten can be used in flavorings in only two instances. One is in hydrolyzed proteins, but with current labeling laws, wheat has to be declared on the label if it's used. The other is in barley malt extract or syrup, but Case points out that it's almost always listed on the label as "barley malt," "barley malt extract," or "barley malt flavoring." She notes that some companies may list it as "flavor (contains barley malt)," but very rarely is it listed as only "flavor" or "natural flavor." So why do I still leave it on the "to be questioned" list? Because "very rarely" leaves room for the possibility, however slight, that barley malt may have been used and listed only as a "flavoring."

Knowing which foods to research

Ingredients you need to question include

- ✔ Brown rice syrup
- ✔ Fillers
- ✔ Flavors and natural flavorings
- ✔ Seasonings and spice blends
- ✔ Stabilizers
- ✔ Starch (in pharmaceuticals)

These ingredients don't always have gluten. In fact, they rarely do. But according to the U.S. Food and Drug Administration Code of Federal Regulations, they *can* contain gluten, so to be safe, you need to check.

Thanks to relatively new labeling laws, far fewer "questionable" ingredients exist because manufacturers now have to clearly indicate whether a product has wheat in it.

Putting an end to the controversy over certain foods

People used to question certain ingredients because of rumors, bad information, misunderstandings, and ambiguous labeling laws. But today, thanks to new labeling laws and more definitive research, the following ingredients are no longer in question:

- ✔ Alcohol (distilled)
- ✔ Caramel color
- ✔ Citric acid
- ✔ Dextrin
- ✔ Flavoring extracts
- ✔ Hydrolyzed plant protein (HPP)
- ✔ Hydrolyzed vegetable protein (HVP)
- ✔ Maltodextrin (except in pharmaceuticals)
- ✔ Modified food starch
- ✔ Mono- and diglycerides
- ✔ Starch (in food)
- ✔ Vanilla and vanilla extract
- ✔ Vinegar (except malt vinegar)
- ✔ Wheat grass
- ✔ Yeast (except brewer's yeast)

 The gluten-free status of these ingredients applies to ingredients produced in the United States and Canada. Other countries may have different manufacturing processes.

The Buzz on Booze: Choosing Alcoholic Beverages

At nearly every talk I give, I'm about five minutes into explaining the diet when someone shoots his hand up Arnold Horshack–style, with a please-tell-me-it-ain't-so look on his face, and I can predict the question: "Beer doesn't have gluten in it . . . does it?" Yeah, it does.

Just a few types of alcoholic beverages aren't allowed on the gluten-free diet. They include (but may not be limited to) the following:

- ✔ Beer (with a few exceptions, such as Budweiser's gluten-free Redbridge beer)
- ✔ Distilled spirits that are added back to the mash
- ✔ Malt beverages

But lots of alcoholic beverages are gluten-free, including

- ✔ Bourbon
- ✔ Brandy
- ✔ Cider (occasionally contains barley, so be careful)
- ✔ Cognac
- ✔ Gin
- ✔ Rum
- ✔ Schnapps
- ✔ Tequila
- ✔ Vodka
- ✔ Whiskey (such as Crown Royal and Jack Daniels)
- ✔ Wine (and sparkling wine or Champagne)

Knowing what kinds of liquor you can consume can be confusing because some alcoholic beverages are distilled from gluten-containing grains. However, as long as the drinks are distilled and the grains aren't added back into the gluten-containing mash, the drinks remain gluten-free.

Making Sure Your Medications and Supplements Are Safe

Anything you ingest can cause problems if it's not gluten-free — even a tiny little pill. Be sure to check the label first because some products actually say "gluten-free" right on the label.

 Starch and modified food starch in pharmaceuticals may come from wheat. If you see either of these on the label, you need to call the manufacturer and find out more about where the starch is from.

If you're wondering about a prescription drug, ask the pharmacist whether the product is gluten-free. If he or she doesn't know, ask for the package insert and use the pharmacy's *Physician's Desk Reference* (the Canadian version of this is called the Compendium of Pharmaceutical Specialties) to look up the name and phone number of the manufacturer. Then you can just call the manufacturer and find out.

 Here are some other ways to ensure your medications are safe for consumption:

✔ Have your pharmacist make a notation in the computer, either under your personal records or under the record for that drug, indicating whether the product is gluten-free.

✔ If the product is over-the-counter, call the manufacturer to confirm the drug's gluten-free status.

✔ Write "GF" in permanent marker on the medica-
tion container so you don't have to wonder
whether the drug is safe when you need to take it.

Using Nonfood Products: What You Need to Know

If you're not eating it, does it really matter whether an
object you use has gluten in it? The answer is this:
sometimes yes and sometimes no. You don't have to
worry about plastic storage containers, pots and
pans, envelopes, or stamps. Here's the scoop on the
gluten content of other key nonfood items so you
know what to check out and what you can let slide:

✔ **Dental products:** Most products used in a dentist's office, such as polish and fluoride, are
gluten-free, but call your dentist in advance and
ask him or her to check for you. As for toothpaste
or mouthwash, I've never found one that contains
gluten, but always read labels just in case.

✔ **External products:** Experts assert that the gluten
molecule is too large to pass through skin, so
lotions, shampoos, conditioners, and other external products shouldn't be a problem unless you
have open sores, rashes, or dermatitis herpetifor-
mis (also known as DH). Then again, if an external product bothers you, don't use it.

Fair warning — sometimes lotion from your
hands or arms can get on the food you're eating
or preparing, and that can cause a problem. Be
sure to wash your hands well (along with any
other area that may touch food) so you don't
end up eating your lotion.

✔ **Makeup:** The makeup that matters most is makeup you're likely to get in your mouth (or someone else's), such as lipstick, lip gloss, lip balm, and lip liner. Foundation, eye shadow, mascara, powder, and other makeup products shouldn't matter unless you get them close to your mouth and could possibly ingest them.

Play-Doh has gluten in it. I know you're not supposed to eat Play-Doh, but really — who can resist a nibble or two? Lots of recipes for gluten-free play-doughs are available from a quick search on the Internet.

Chapter 4

Shopping Is Easier Than You Think

· ·

In This Chapter

▶ Developing strategies before you head to the store

▶ Figuring out what you want to buy

▶ Exploring your options of stores and more

▶ Getting the most for your gluten-free dollar

· ·

*F*inding gluten-free products really *is* easier than you may think, and thanks to improved labeling laws and manufacturer awareness, it's getting easier all the time. In this chapter, I help you figure out what you want to buy and offer some guidance on where and how to shop and how to save money on gluten-free foods.

Knowing What You Want

One of the best things you can do to make shopping easier when you're enjoying a gluten-free lifestyle is plan ahead. If you try to wing it, especially at first, you end up spending hours in the grocery store walking in circles, trying to figure out what to eat and what to buy, and *then* worrying about whether the food's gluten-free.

Not only do planning meals ahead of time and making shopping lists save you time and head-aches in the store but these steps also give you the peace of mind that the meals you're plan-ning are, in fact, gluten-free.

Planning your meals

In my other life, when I'm a businesswoman and not an author, I follow the dictum *plan your work and work your plan.* Same thing goes for meals, although *plan your meals and eat 'em* isn't quite as catchy or clever.

Most people think planning meals sounds like a great idea, and they're able to pull it off once or twice. But for the most part, they're spontaneous and impulsive. They see something in the store that looks particu-larly appealing (and because they're usually starving while they're shopping, *everything* looks good), and they toss it in the cart. But planning meals helps you strategize before you head to the store.

When you're planning your meals, try not to think in terms of cutting out gluten. Instead, think of how you can make substitutions. Think about the things you love to eat — with or with-out gluten — and build around those foods, making the substitutions you need to make to convert gluten-containing meals into gluten-free ones. (In Chapter 5, I explain how to make *any-thing* gluten-free with simple substitutions.)

I know, sitting down and making a meal plan is tough, but it pays off in spades when you're at the store and you find your busy weekdays speeding by. You may find some of these tips helpful:

✔ **Have the whole family eat gluten-free.** Even if some members of your family are still gluten-eaters, make your life simpler by planning most, if not all, of the family meals to be gluten-free. This planning isn't hard if you follow the *if man made it, don't eat it* approach of eating meats, fruits, vegetables, and other natural foods. And even if your meal includes things like pasta, the gluten-free varieties these days are so delicious that the entire family will love them — and may not even know the difference.

✔ **Plan a few days' menus at once.** Look through cookbooks (they don't have to be gluten-free ones) or at individual recipes for inspiration. Remember, the gluten-free diet is *not* all about rice, corn, and potatoes. In fact, the more variety, the better. Variety isn't just the spice of life; it's important from a nutritional standpoint. Rice, corn, and potatoes don't offer much nutritionally. Try the more nutritious foods I talk about in Chapter 3, such as quinoa and millet.

✔ **Plan a marathon cooking day.** Maybe you designate Sundays to be your day in the kitchen. With the week's worth of meals already in mind, you can prepare several meals at once, saving yourself time shopping, cooking, *and* cleaning up during the week. Because you'll have menu ideas fresh in your hand and food won't go to waste, you'll probably save money, too.

✔ **Use foods that can do double-duty.** If you're planning to cook a large roasting chicken for dinner one night, you can count on leftovers for chicken stir-fry the next night.

✔ **Plan meals you can cook in a slow cooker.** Slow cookers are great for complete one-course meals. Plus, walking into a house that smells like you've been cooking all day is a great way to say "welcome home!"

Have the whole family help with menu planning. Nothing is more frustrating than spending a weekend planning, shopping, and cooking only to hear moans and groans about how what used to be someone's favorite food is now "gross." Let them offer suggestions — for that matter, enlist help with the cooking and cleanup, too.

Making lists

Shopping lists not only remind you of the foods and ingredients you need but they also help prevent impulse shopping. How many times have you roamed the grocery store thinking of yummy, healthy meals to make for the week, only to get home with dozens of bags of groceries, unable to remember a single meal? Yeah, me too. Your spontaneity is exactly what food manufacturers are banking on, which is why they tempt you with the delicious-but-oh-so-bad-for-you, high-profit-margin foods at the ends of aisles and checkout stands. A shopping list is your key to foiling their plan.

Keep a list of what you're running low on or what you need to buy the next time you're at the store. Make sure the list is handy for everyone in the family so no one whines that you "forgot" a favorite food (when you didn't even know that *was* a favorite food).

As you do your menu planning, add the ingredients you need for your week's worth of meals to the list. If you need to call manufacturers to find out whether some of the ingredients are gluten-free, now's the best time to do so (if the product's not sitting in front of you, you can usually find the manufacturer's phone number online). Don't wait until you're in the store, because you may find that the company's customer service representatives have all gone home for the day. Oh, and don't forget to take the list with you (that's a note to myself, because I usually forget it)!

 If you're a coupon-clipper, clip your coupons and refer to your grocery list and the store ads. Can you replace items on your list with ones that are on sale or that you have coupons for? You may even find that the coupons provide inspiration for meal planning. Just be careful not to buy things simply *because* you have coupons; instead, use your coupons only for things you really need.

 Don't forget the snacks! Whether your idea of a snack is ice cream or raisins, snacks are an important part of your day. When you're making your shopping list, encourage your family members to add their favorite snacks — preferably the healthy kind — so you don't have to hear "there's nothing to eat in this house!"

Deciding What to Buy

Obviously, the most important considerations for figuring out what to buy are what you like, what you're going to make, and whether it's gluten-free.

Keep in mind the two kinds of gluten-free foods: foods that companies make as specialty items and foods that are naturally gluten-free.

Checking out gluten-free specialty products

Gluten-free specialty items come from companies that specifically market some or all of their products to the wheat-free/gluten-free community. Most of the time, these products are foods that would normally have gluten in them — such as pasta, bread, crackers, cookies, and brownies — but have been formulated to be gluten-free.

The specialty products are almost always labeled *gluten-free,* so you don't have to question their safety as far as your dietary restrictions are concerned. The companies that make these products generally make several product lines and sell their foods by mail, online, or at specialty retailers. These days, "regular" grocery stores are starting to carry more of these specialty items.

 Wheat has to be called out on the label, so it's pretty easy to avoid. But remember that *wheat-free* doesn't mean *gluten-free.* If you see a package labeled *wheat-free,* the contents may still contain barley, rye, oats, or derivatives of those ingredients. Read the label carefully to see whether it lists other forms of gluten besides wheat.

Remembering naturally gluten-free foods

Many people think the gluten-free lifestyle limits them to buying foods that say *gluten-free* on the label. This is *so* not true! Limiting yourself to those foods is ultra-restrictive, and it also means you're overlooking lots of foods that are naturally gluten-free, some of which are the most nutritious of all. These are foods that contain no gluten, although the distributor doesn't necessarily market them as such. They include the obvious players — meat, poultry, fish, seafood, fruits, vegetables, and nuts — but they also include some products that seem like they may have gluten in them but don't.

Many foods, including most candies, chips, popcorn, deli foods, condiments, and spices, are naturally gluten-free. Even some commercial cereals are gluten-free but aren't labeled as such.

Asian foods — such as rice wraps, many Thai dishes, and most fish or oyster sauces — are good examples of foods that are often naturally gluten-free (remember, though, that soy sauce usually has wheat in it). Mexican and other ethnic cuisines also offer a lot of inherently gluten-free foods. So although they don't say *gluten-free* on the label, they are, in fact, often safe on the gluten-free diet.

> The best foods are those without a label: meat, seafood, produce, and so on. But many other foods are gluten-free and don't say so on the label. Read the list of ingredients, and if you don't see anything blatantly off-limits, call the manufacturer to confirm that the food is gluten-free. You'll be surprised at how often you find products that you can safely enjoy.

Asking for opinions

The last thing you want to do is spend gobs of money on specialty items and expensive foods only to find that they taste more like cardboard than cake. Because gluten-free foods can be pricey, and because some are great and some are awful, asking around about gluten-free foods and getting opinions from others who've tried them is more important than ever. Of course, opinions vary, and what one person loves, another may hate, but opinions can be valuable, especially if you hear several of them.

> If you want to hear opinions on products, you have a lot of options. Try some of these places:

✔ **Support groups:** If you attend support group meetings, ask the members whether they've ever tried a particular product or whether they have suggestions for, say, brownies. You can get lots of helpful ideas this way.

✔ **Listservs:** You can subscribe to these free e-mail lists. Posting questions and comments about gluten-free products is a valuable part of belonging to a listserv.

✔ **Online rating systems:** Some of the online shopping Web sites offer customer ratings. See how many stars a product has and read the comments to help you decide whether you want to buy it.

✔ **Shoppers:** If you see people at a store buying a product you haven't tried, ask whether they've tried it and what they like or don't like about it. At the same time, if you've tried a product and see someone looking at it, speak up. He or she will appreciate the input, I assure you.

✔ **Store staff:** Sometimes the store staff members are very knowledgeable about products. Ask them whether they've tried a particular product and what they like or don't like about it. Be careful, though — sometimes a staffer sounds knowledgeable but isn't. Make sure you know your facts well enough to tell the difference.

When you find products that you and your family love and have confirmed to be gluten-free, save the label or part of the packaging. Keep the labels in a binder and create divided sections such as "Soup," "Candy," or whatever category you like. Then, bring the binder with you to the store so you can quickly spot the items again and rest easy knowing that you like the product and that it is, in fact, gluten-free.

Deciding Where to Shop

So you know what meals you want to make, you have at least some idea of what foods you want to buy, and you may even have a list in hand. Where do you get all this stuff (some of which you've never heard of)? Well, for most of your shopping needs, you can pick a store — any store — because you're not as limited as you may think. The next sections list your many options.

"Regular" grocery stores

You can do most of your shopping at "regular" grocery stores — yep, the kind you find on every corner in most cities. If you're surprised by this, don't be. Remember, I encourage you to eat mostly foods that are naturally healthy and inherently gluten-free, and you can find those at your friendly neighborhood grocery store.

Obviously, these stores are more convenient and less expensive than specialty stores. But from a psychological standpoint, you have a couple of other, less tangible reasons for shopping at a regular grocery store.

First, a gluten-free diet can seem restrictive and even daunting to some people, and some even find it to be somewhat isolating (although hopefully not after they're finished with *this* book). Being forced to shop only at specialty stores or online confirms those feelings of isolation and despair. Being able to shop at "regular" stores and buy "regular" brands that everyone else is buying is really liberating for people who feel this way.

If you have kids on the gluten-free diet, considering the psychological impact of shopping at regular grocery stores is even more important. Kids want to be like all the other kids and eat brands (and junk foods) that all the other kids eat. And that's okay — feeling that way is perfectly normal. For most kids, fitting in ranks right up there with breathing. Shopping at "regular" grocery stores gives them the sense of normalcy that they crave.

Regular brands aside, many major grocery stores are starting to carry more gluten-free specialty items; some even have entire gluten-free sections. If you have some favorite specialty products that you want your local store to carry, don't hesitate to ask the manager whether the store can carry them. How often you get a positive response may surprise you, and the manager may be surprised at how much interest customers have in the gluten-free products.

You may also be pleased to know that many of the regular grocery chains have lists of the gluten-free products they carry, both name brand and generic. Some of the stores post the lists on their Web sites, and others offer the lists if you call their customer service numbers.

Natural foods stores

Most natural foods stores are well aware of the growing interest in gluten-free products, and they're stocking up to meet the increasing demand. You can find all the meats and vegetables (usually organic) that are such a big part of the gluten-free diet, but you can also find lots of gluten-free specialty items. Some natural foods stores even have dedicated gluten-free sections.

Because natural foods stores have become so popular, they've expanded their offerings and generally provide a huge array of exotic and gourmet health foods, supplements, and even cosmetics and household goods. Shopping at some of these places is more like being in a fun zone than a food zone.

Farmers' markets

Farmers' markets are popping up everywhere (not just next to farms), offering fresh produce, eggs, meat, fish, honey, nuts, and other (naturally gluten-free) items, usually at prices far below those of most retailers. The foods are ripe, organic is the rule rather than the exception, and the generous samples that sellers pass out are enough to count as lunch.

You can also feel good knowing you're supporting local farmers and the environment: The food is usually grown without pesticides, and not having to ship the foods long distances uses less energy and gasoline.

Ethnic markets

You want a gluten-free kind of a thrill? Go to an Asian market — the more authentic, the better — and check out all the stuff that's gluten-free. Don't forget the Thai and Indian aisles. Truly, the selection is amazing. Sauces, rice wraps, tapioca noodles, rice candies, things you've never heard of, and things that you may wonder about for years — all gluten-free. Of course, they're not labeled as such, but that's okay. If the label is in English, you can see for yourself that gluten isn't in many of the foods. Asians use very little wheat in their products.

Other ethnic cuisines may surprise and delight as well. Mexican is just one of the many other cultures that use lots of inherently gluten-free ingredients in their cooking. Explore new cultures without ever leaving your country and experience a thrill of the gluten-free variety.

Gluten-free retail stores

I'm not making this up. Once only a dream for those who've been gluten-free for a long time, gluten-free stores are finally a reality. Entire stores filled with gluten-free foods, books about being gluten-free, cookbooks, and other important resources are beginning to pop up, and I'm delighted to say they're thriving. You'll be seeing more and more of these, so keep your eyes peeled for a store opening near you.

Web sites and catalogs

You can do all of your gluten-free shopping from the comfort of your favorite easy chair, any time, day or night — you can even be in your comfiest jammies, if you want. Some great Web sites specialize in selling gluten-free products, and within just a few minutes, you can place your order. A couple of days later, your shipment arrives at your doorstep — and you may be so excited to rip open that big box of gluten-free goodies that you feel like a kid at the holidays!

 All the gluten-free specialty food manufacturers have Web sites, so if you know a specific brand you want to buy, you can go to the site and see what they have to offer (you can find the sites with a quick Google search). But here are a couple sites you can buy several different brands from:

✔ www.glutenfreemall.com

✔ www.glutenfree.com

✔ www.amazon.com (search under "Grocery" for gluten-free)

If you don't have a computer, most companies offer a toll-free number, and some will send you a free catalog so you can order by phone or fax.

Navigating the Aisles

For decades now, grocery store psychologists have been studying ways to get people to spend more, and they've come up with subtle and subliminal ways to turn us all into Stepford Shoppers, falling victim to strategically placed temptations scattered about the store like land mines.

One of the best ways to avoid some of those glaring gluten temptations at the store is to shop the perimeter. Store layouts are predictable; produce, dairy, meat, and other staples are as far from the front door of the store as possible so that you have to walk past all the more expensive (and usually less nutritious) foods before you get to what you really want. By sticking to the perimeter for most things, you can save yourself a lot of time by not having to go through the cracker, cookie, and bread aisles.

Copy a safe and forbidden ingredients list off the Internet (try the "Safe Gluten-Free Food List/ Unsafe Foods & Ingredients" link at www.celiac. com) and bring it with you to the store. You may need it when you're reading ingredients on product labels.

Living Gluten-Free — Affordably

One of the most common complaints I hear about the gluten-free diet is that it's more expensive — but it doesn't need to be. Yes, I understand that a loaf of regular bread is less than half the cost of a loaf of gluten-free bread. And the fact that gluten-free crackers and cookies are often smaller *and* twice the price of regular cookies isn't lost on me, either. And yes, I've paid more than my fair share in shipping expenses. But you have ways to save significant amounts of money when you're enjoying a gluten-free lifestyle. So before you take a second mortgage on your house to finance this diet, take note of these tips that can save you a bunch.

Scaling back on specialties

Most of the "extra expense" of the gluten-free diet is in the high cost of specialty items. I'm not suggesting you celebrate little Preston's birthday with store-bought rice crackers to save the expense of making a gluten-free cake. You need to have *some* specialty items on hand, and cakes or special-occasion treats are definitely among them.

But if you find you're spending way too much money to accommodate this diet, take a look at how many and what types of specialty items you buy. Breads, crackers, cookies, cakes, pizzas, pretzels, donuts — they're pricey, for sure. But you don't need them. You can substitute store-bought chips for a fraction of the cost of gluten-free pretzels. Even as high-priced as they are, candies and candy bars that you can get at any grocery store are far cheaper than specialty treats.

And really, most of the specialty items aren't good for you, anyway — they're high-calorie, they raise your blood sugar quickly, and they provide very little nutritional value.

Some of the specialty items people buy are unnecessary. Gluten-free vanilla is a good example: All vanilla is gluten-free! You don't need to buy it as a specialty item.

Some specialty items may be important to have on hand — pasta, some special-occasion treats, and maybe some bread or bagels, for instance. But in general, most people buy more specialty items than they need, and it definitely puts a burden on the budget.

Tax deductions for the gluten-free

Believe it or not, there's a tax deduction available when you buy gluten-free food, but not everyone can take advantage of it. You can deduct the *difference* in price between gluten-free products and "regular" food products. Here's an example using a loaf of bread:

Gluten-free bread: $5.00

"Regular" bread: $2.00

Difference in price: $3.00

You can deduct the $3.00 difference. The cost of items you wouldn't normally need to buy, like xanthan gum, are completely deductible. Shipping costs are deductible, too. But to qualify, your unreimbursed medical expenses must exceed 7.5 percent of your adjusted gross income. That's a pretty tall order for most people. You also need a letter from your doctor saying that a gluten-free diet is medically necessary for you. All of these expenses are reimbursable under a health care spending account of pretax income. Consult a tax advisor for more information.

Saving on shipping

If you do buy specialty items, you can find ways to save on shipping. For one, you can ask your local grocery or natural foods store to carry the product you want — that way the store pays for the shipping, not you.

If you're ordering online, order from a company that sells many different brands of products. That way you pay one shipping charge for several different brands. (Buying one or two products at a time from individual manufacturers costs you a fortune in shipping.)

Going generic

Don't assume that generics are off-limits on a gluten-free diet. Most of the time, generic products are as clearly labeled as major brands, and sometimes a toll-free number is listed on the package so you can call to confirm whether the item is gluten-free. Usually, generics are labeled as being *distributed by* a large grocery chain or distribution company. Dig a little — call toll-free information or go on the Internet to get a phone number for the large grocery chain or distribution company. Most of the time, you can locate a customer service representative who can help you find out more about the ingredients.

If the generics are a store brand, chances are good that you'll be able to get lots of information about the products. Some of the large grocery chains have lists of their gluten-free generics, and sometimes those lists are even available online. If you want more information about a store's generic products, call its toll-free number and ask to talk with the head of quality control or the nutrition department. I did this once and was pleased to hear from the lead nutritionist that the modified food starch in all of their generic products was derived from corn. That little bit of information was immensely helpful in realizing that even more generics than I'd known were gluten-free.

Eating nutritiously

Some people think that eating nutritious foods is more expensive. Not true. Fresh produce and meats do seem expensive — they are! But chips and other processed, blood-sugar-raising foods — which not only are worthless nutritionally but also cause weight gain and make you hungrier — are a complete waste of money.

Buy nutritious foods, but buy only what you need. Most nutritious foods are also perishable, and if you don't use them within a few days, fresh produce isn't so fresh anymore.

Eating in

Eating out at restaurants or fast-food places eats through a budget in no time. Eating at home not only ensures that your meal is, in fact, gluten-free but it also saves you money.

Sure, planning and preparing home-cooked meals takes time (I give some time-saving tips in Chapter 5), but the money you save and the peace of mind you get knowing that your meals are nutritious and gluten-free are well worth it.

Using gluten-free mixes

The gluten-free mixes for baked goods such as brownies, cakes, cookies, and breads may seem expensive, and they are. But compare them to the cost of buying several different types of specialty flours, xanthan gum (a must-have in gluten-free baking recipes), and other ingredients you need to make those homemade baked goods, and then add on the cost of the failed attempts (you *will* have some failures). Suddenly, the surefire-taste-delicious-and-always-turn-out-right mixes seem like a bargain.

Developing good shopping habits

In addition to what I cover in this chapter, you can do a lot to save time and money when you shop. Here's a list to get you started:

✔ **Don't shop when you're hungry.** If you shop on an empty stomach, you're more vulnerable to impulse purchases.

✔ **Stock up when you can to save cash.** Remember, though, that gluten-free foods often have a short shelf life. Make sure you have room in your freezer.

✔ **Join membership clubs.** Membership clubs are usually the big warehouse-type stores. These stores are especially good if you want to buy in bulk because most of their products are supersized.

✔ **Use coupons, flyers, rebates, and frequent-shopper programs.** You can save hundreds of dollars a year by taking advantage of product incentives. Even if you're a less-than-enthusiastic coupon clipper, try to find a few to use each week and don't forget to check the circulars that are at the front of the stores.

✔ **Dare to compare.** Always look at the unit price of a product, not just the package price, so that when you're comparing the price of one item to another, you're comparing apples to apples.

✔ **Watch to make sure the scanner rings up the correct price.** Stores do make mistakes, and a lot of times those mistakes aren't in your favor.

✔ **If possible, don't shop with your kids.** Grocery stores are counting on your kids to lure you into impulsive purchases of high-profit-margin treats like cereals and snack foods.

Chapter 5

Cooking Tips and Techniques

. . . .

In This Chapter

▶ Embracing creativity in your gluten-free cooking

▶ Putting wheat alternatives to work

▶ Entering the wonderful world of gluten-free baking

. . . .

I have some unique cooking tips and techniques that can help in your gluten-free cooking adventures, and I cover them in this chapter. If you know me or have watched me cook, I'm sure you're smirking right now because the truth of the matter is that I have a — ahem — *different* style of cooking, and you're probably wondering what I'm doing giving cooking tips. I don't want to point fingers, but my editors made me do it! Somehow they didn't think "open bag of mix, approximate measurements, and improvise" would sit well with anyone who wants to do real cooking.

Don't get me wrong. I love to cook. But I do it my way. My measuring terms consist of *dollop, gob,* and *itsy bit,* and I use them interchangeably. If you like the more technical approach, that's okay. I had a real, live cookbook author write the recipes for my gluten-free cookbook, *Gluten-Free Cooking For Dummies* (I wrote the nonrecipe part of it, and it's published by Wiley). But if you prefer to cook without the safety net of recipes, you're still okay. The tips and techniques in this chapter apply to you whether you're my kind of cook or of the more scrupulous variety.

Creatively Gluten-Free: Improvising in the Kitchen

Basically, I follow a few simple rules of cooking:

- ✔ Measuring is for patient people. I don't qualify.

- ✔ If a recipe calls for ¼ teaspoon of something, why bother?

- ✔ If a recipe calls for more than 12 ingredients, and if I have to go to a foreign country to purchase any of them, I don't bother.

- ✔ What's a sifter for?

- ✔ If you bake it in your oven, it *is* homemade. Therefore, by definition, using mixes qualifies as homemade cooking.

I believe that if you give a person a recipe, you feed him for a meal; teach him to make recipes gluten-free, and you feed him for a lifetime. I also think finding out how to improvise and cook *anything* gluten-free has a lot of value. Sometimes that means modifying a recipe for something that normally has gluten in it so that it's gluten-free. Other times that means throwing caution to the wind and doing without a recipe altogether.

No single ingredient is more important in gluten-free cooking than creativity. You may not always have ingredients on hand to make the gluten-free dish you want to make. You may not have a recipe handy for a meal you have in mind. You may think you have no way to convert your old favorite standby into a gluten-free goodie. Don't let any of those things stop you. Cooking gluten-free is actually easy if you improvise, explore alternatives, and stretch the boundaries of your creativity in the kitchen. The following sections help you do just that by showing you how to adapt non-gluten-free recipes, avoid cross-contamination, and make delicious substitutions.

Adapting any dish to be gluten-free

You can modify nearly any dish to be gluten-free. Some dishes are easier than others — baked goods are the toughest, so I deal with those last. You can go one of two ways when you're adapting a dish to be gluten-free: with a recipe or without.

- ✔ **If you're following a recipe for something that's not gluten-free and you want to convert it, start by reviewing the list of ingredients the recipe calls for.** Make a note of those that usually have gluten in them. Then, using the substitutions I suggest in this chapter or some of your own, substitute gluten-free ingredients as you need to. (For the most part, when you make substitutions, measurements convert equally — with the exception of flours, as you find out in the later "Substituting gluten-free flours" section.)

  Don't have the right substitutions? Improvise. For instance, if a recipe calls for dredging something in flour before sautéing and you don't have any gluten-free flours, maybe you have a gluten-free mix that would work. Pancake mix or even muffin mix can work quite well as a substitute for a flour coating.

- ✔ **If you're not using a recipe, let creativity prevail.** Say you want to make chicken nuggets. You certainly don't need a recipe for that; just slice some chicken and figure out what you want to coat it in before frying or baking. Put some of your favorite gluten-free barbecue potato chips in a plastic bag and crunch them up. Now you have a coating!

Avoiding cross-contamination when cooking

After you've worked hard to create a delicious gluten-free meal, you wouldn't go dust a bunch of wheat flour all over it, would you? Of course not. Yet sometimes the *way* you cook food can contaminate it as though you had done just that, and you may not be aware that your food is being contaminated.

 Cooking gluten-containing foods at the same time as gluten-free ones is okay, but be aware that cross-contamination during the cooking process is a very real consideration. Be careful not to *glutenate* (contaminate with gluten) your food inadvertently. Watch out for these pitfalls:

✔ **Cooking utensils:** You can't flip a gluten-containing hamburger bun with a spatula and then flip a burger. Well, you can, but that burger is no longer gluten-free. Same thing goes for tossing the pasta and stirring the sauce. Use separate utensils while you're cooking and keep track of which one is which.

✔ **Double-duty cooking surfaces:** If you're cooking gluten-containing and gluten-free foods on the same griddle, grills, or cookie sheets or in the same pans, cook the gluten-free version first. If that just doesn't work, you can use the same cooking surface for both versions, but be sure to find a clean spot for your gluten-free foods.

✔ **Frying oil:** When you fry breaded products in oil, bits of the breading or batter stay in the oil when you're finished frying. So if you fry gluten-containing foods in oil, don't use that same oil to fry your gluten-free foods. Either fry the gluten-free foods first or use completely separate pans and fresh oil for the gluten-free foods.

If you're cooking both glutenous and gluten-free foods in your fryer, you'll need to be extra diligent when you're cleaning it to make sure you get all the gluten out. If your fryer isn't easy to clean thoroughly, you may want to consider having separate fryers.

Using standby substitutions

To convert a recipe that usually contains gluten into one that's gluten-free, you need to make some simple substitutions. For the most part, with the exception of flours you use when making baked goods, the substitutions are simple — just swap one for the other. (I cover flours for baked goods later in this chapter.)

- ✔ **Beer:** Some foods, especially deep-fried foods, may call for beer in the recipe. You can either use the gluten-free beers available online or try cider instead.

- ✔ **Binders:** A *binder* is just something that holds foodstuff together. Because gluten provides elasticity and stretch to baked goods, adding binders to foods that don't have gluten-containing flours in them is a good idea. Binders include xanthan gum, guar gum, gelatin powder (which adds protein and moisture), and eggs.

- ✔ **Breadcrumbs:** No-brainer here. Anyone who's ever eaten a piece of gluten-free bread (especially without toasting it) knows that breadcrumbs aren't hard to come by. You can buy gluten-free breadcrumbs from specialty stores or online, but if you can't or don't want to get those, consider using any gluten-free bread. Just put the bread in a plastic bag and smoosh it into the size of crumbs you want. You can even toast the crumbs if you want added crunch or need dry breadcrumbs rather than fresh ones. Crushed cereals work well in place of breadcrumbs, too. Also consider using mashed potato flakes or quinoa flakes.

✔ **Bun:** Consider using a lettuce wrap, corn tortilla, or, of course, gluten-free bread. Some good gluten-free buns are available online and at specialty shops.

✔ **Coatings:** If a recipe calls for some type of coating, you have several options. You can despair and not make the dish (kidding!), or you can consider using any of the gluten-free flours I list later in this chapter, as well as any versatile gluten-free mix you have lying around, such as a mix for bread, muffins, or pancakes. Cornmeal or corn flour *(masa)* with seasonings mixed in adds an interesting texture, and crushed barbecue potato chips (gluten-free, of course) are one of my personal all-time favorites. You may also want to look into commercial brands of Cajun-style coatings, which are usually marketed as seafood seasonings. Many of those are just cornmeal with some spices added.

✔ **"Cream of" soups:** Use chicken broth and sour cream or half-and-half. If you're going for ultra-nutritious, blend cooked cauliflower in the blender and use that for the "cream of" part. Remember to add the food the soup is a cream of — mushroom, celery, potato, and so on — to complete it.

✔ **Croutons:** Homemade croutons are actually very easy to make. Cut fresh gluten-free bread into the size cubes you want and deep-fry them. After you drain and cool them, roll them in

Parmesan cheese, spices, or any other flavoring you like.

✔ **Fillers:** *Filler* is a highly technical culinary term for something that fills stuff in. Yum. Generally not something you hope to see on a label, fillers aren't always a bad thing; they may be in meatloaf, for example, where the recipe often calls for breadcrumbs, crackers, and other filler-type materials to add, well, filling. Gluten-free bread or breadcrumbs provides an obvious substitution here, but also consider leftover corn bread, mashed potato flakes, or even an unsweetened cereal that you've crushed up.

✔ **Flour:** Many recipes call for flour, usually to serve as a thickener (see the suggested thickeners in this list). Also consider using gluten-free flours such as rice flour, sweet rice flour (they're different), potato starch, sorghum flour, garbanzo/fava bean flour, and Montina (Indian ricegrass flour).

✔ **Flour tortillas:** The obvious substitution here is corn tortillas. Some new gluten-free flour tortillas are on the market now, and you can find recipes for homemade tortillas online or in cookbooks. Other wrap substitutions include rice wraps (found in Asian markets) and lettuce.

✔ **Pie crust:** One of the easiest ways to make a pie crust is to smash your favorite cereal into tiny crumbs, add some butter (and sugar, if the cereal isn't sweet enough), and then press the mixture into the bottom of a pie pan. Some good gluten-free crackers and cookies work well the same way. Some pie crusts are supposed to be cooked before adding the pie filling; others aren't. The fact that the crust is gluten-free doesn't change, regardless of whether you need to cook the crust before filling the pie. Also check out some of the gluten-free pie crust mixes available on the Internet and at specialty stores.

✔ **Sandwich squeezers:** These items are what are otherwise known as the bread "ends" of a sandwich, and you have lots of alternatives to bread. Try a lettuce wrap, corn tortilla, waffle, or pancake (the toaster-oven variety is great for this). Of course, gluten-free bread works too, if you can find a variety you like.

✔ **Soy sauce:** Most soy sauce has wheat in it (and the label clearly indicates wheat), but you can find brands that are wheat-free. (By the way, *tamari* — a thicker, Japanese soy sauce — isn't always wheat-free, so check the label.) Either use a wheat-free soy sauce or try Bragg Liquid Aminos. You may also want to get adventurous and try an Asian sauce like fish sauce (careful — it's really fishy!) or oyster sauce.

✔ **Teriyaki:** Because most soy sauce has wheat in it, most teriyaki (which is made from soy sauce) does too. A few brands of wheat-free teriyaki sauces are available, but don't be afraid to make your own (see my recipe in the nearby "Making teriyaki sauce" sidebar).

✔ **Thickeners:** Many recipes call for flour as a thickener, but lots of alternatives are available. For sweet things, try using a dry pudding mix or gelatin. ClearJel works well with acidic ingredients (unlike cornstarch), tolerates high temperatures, and doesn't cause pie fillings to "weep" during storage. Arrowroot flour, agar, tapioca starch, and cornstarch are also excellent thickeners. So is sweet rice flour, which comes from sticky or glutinous rice (despite the name, it really is gluten-free). And remember that muffin or cake mix you have lying around. Not only do mixes thicken the recipe, but the sweet flavor is a pleasant surprise.

Making teriyaki sauce

Actually, the term *teriyaki* refers to a method of cooking, derived from the Japanese words *teri,* meaning "luster," and *yaki,* meaning "grill" or "broil" (cleverly combined to form the word *teriyaki*). Traditional teriyaki dishes are marinated in the sauce and then grilled or broiled, creating a shiny *(teri)* glaze. Although you can substitute for it, the key ingredient in teriyaki sauce is *mirin,* a sweet Japanese rice wine used for cooking. To make your own teriyaki sauce, use the following ingredients:

✔ ½ cup soy sauce

✔ ½ cup mirin (**Note:** If you don't have mirin, use ½ cup sake and 1 tablespoon sugar.)

✔ 3 tablespoons sugar

In a small saucepan, mix together the soy sauce, mirin, and sugar. Heat on low heat for about 3 minutes and then let the sauce cool. You can store teriyaki sauce in a clean bottle in the fridge.

Cooking with Wheat Alternatives

Most gluten-free cooking is pretty straightforward and isn't much different from "regular" cooking if you let your creative side take over. You just substitute gluten-free ingredients for the gluten-containing ones and, for the most part, you're set. (**Note:** The process is a little different for baked goods, as I explain later in this chapter.) I show you the ins and outs of using gluten-free grains, starches, and flours in the next sections.

Incorporating alternative gluten-free grains

Not only are the gluten-free grains and grain alternatives that I talk about in Chapter 3 ultra-nutritious, but they add unique flavors and textures to foods, too. For the most part, cooking them is just like cooking other grains, but you do need to know a few things to perfect the art of using alternative gluten-free grains.

When cooking gluten-free grains as whole grains (as opposed to using them as a flour in baked goods), you find that these alternative grains cook like most whole grains — just toss them in boiling water, reduce the heat so the water simmers, and you're set. The grain-to-water proportion and cooking times are really the only things that vary. Table 5-1 has some approximations of amounts of liquids and cooking times; you can modify them to suit your preferences.

Table 5-1	Cooking Alternative Grains	
Gluten-Free Grain (1 Cup)	*Amount of Water or Chicken Broth*	*Cooking Time*
Amaranth	2½ cups	20 to 25 minutes
Brown rice (long or short grain)	3 cups	40 minutes
Buckwheat	2 cups	15 to 20 minutes
Corn (grits)	3 cups	5 to 10 minutes
Millet	3 cups	35 to 45 minutes
Quinoa	2 cups	15 to 20 minutes
Teff	2 cups	15 to 20 minutes
White rice	2 cups	15 minutes
Wild rice	4 cups	45 minutes

Quinoa, millet, teff, amaranth, buckwheat, and the other alternative grains are great additions to soups, stuffing, and other foods. You can use alternative grains in other places, too, whether you precook them or simply toss them in with the other ingredients.

- ✔ **Snacks:** Using a little oil in a pan, you can pop amaranth grains on the stove like popcorn and eat them seasoned or plain.

- ✔ **Soups:** Use buckwheat, quinoa, or millet in soups instead of rice or noodles. No need to cook the grains first; just add them to the soup as you're cooking it (but remember that they absorb the liquid and double in volume). Whole amaranth and teff are too small, and they may seem gritty in soups, although both work well to thicken soups if you use the flour form of them.

- ✔ **Stuffing:** Use the larger alternative grains, such as cooked quinoa, millet, or buckwheat, instead of breadcrumbs or croutons in stuffing. Season the stuffing to your taste and then stuff vegetables, poultry, or pork tenderloins.

Thickening with gluten-free starches and flours

People usually use starch-based thickeners such as cornstarch, arrowroot, and tapioca to thicken their sauces and gravies. Starch thickeners give food a transparent, glistening sheen, which looks great for pie fillings and in glazes. The thickeners don't always look quite right in gravy or sauce, though, so knowing which ones to use is important.

 To thicken with gluten-free starches, mix the starch with an equal amount of cold liquid until it forms a paste. Then whisk the paste into the liquid you're trying to thicken. After you add the thickener to the liquid, cook it for at least 30 seconds or so to get rid of the starchy flavor. But be careful you don't overcook it — liquids that you thicken with these starches may get thin again if you cook them too long or at too high a temperature.

Some of these flours have the advantage of working well with foods that are acidic. Acidic foods include canned or glazed fruits, citrus, tomatoes, and vinegar. Bananas, figs, avocados, and potatoes are examples of foods that aren't acidic (they're actually alkaline).

Take a look at your options for thickeners:

- ✔ **Arrowroot:** If you're looking for that shiny gloss for dessert sauces or glazes, arrowroot is a good bet. Use arrowroot if you're thickening an acidic liquid but not if you're using dairy products (it makes them slimy). Arrowroot has the most neutral taste of all the starch thickeners, so if you're worried that a thickener may change or mask the flavor of your dish, use arrowroot. You can freeze the sauces you make with arrowroot.

- ✔ **ClearJel:** This modified cornstarch works especially well for fruit pie fillings because it blends well with acidic ingredients, tolerates high temperatures, and doesn't cause pie fillings to "weep" during storage. It also doesn't begin thickening until the liquid begins to cool, which allows the heat to be more evenly distributed within the jar if you're canning.

- ✔ **Cornstarch:** Cornstarch is the best choice for thickening dairy-based sauces, but don't use it for acidic foods. Cornstarch isn't as shiny as tapioca or arrowroot. Don't use cornstarch if you're freezing the sauce, or the sauce will get spongy.

✔ **Potato starch:** Usually used to thicken soups and gravies, potato starch doesn't work well in liquids that you boil. Unlike cornstarch and some other grain-based foods, potato starch is a permitted ingredient for Passover.

✔ **Tapioca:** You can use pearl tapioca or tapioca granules to thicken puddings and pies, but they don't dissolve completely when you cook them, so you end up with tiny gelatinous balls. If you like the balls, you can also use instant tapioca to thicken soups, gravies, and stews. If you don't like them, you can get tapioca starch, which is already finely ground. Tapioca gives a glossy sheen and can tolerate prolonged cooking and freezing.

You can use any of the alternative grains to thicken sauces, gravies, stews, puddings — anything! Depending on what you're making, you can use whole grains or flours as a thickener. You probably want to use a flour instead of whole grain to thicken something like gravy, but whole grains add lots of nutrition and work well to thicken soups and stews.

When you're using the following flours or starches as thickeners, keep in mind that substitution amounts are a little different. Instead of 1 tablespoon of all-purpose flour, use these amounts:

✔ **Agar:** ½ tablespoon

✔ **Arrowroot:** 2 teaspoons

✔ **Cornstarch:** ½ tablespoon

✔ **Gelatin powder:** ½ tablespoon

✔ **Rice flour (brown or white):** 1 tablespoon

✔ **Sweet potato flour:** 1 tablespoon

Trying Your Hand at Gluten-Free Baking

I won't sugarcoat the situation: Baking is the trickiest type of gluten-free cooking you can try. But it's getting easier. Years ago, gluten-free baking produced brick-like breads and cakes that crumbled when you exposed them to air.

Gluten is what makes baked goods stretchy, elastic, and doughy. It also forms a support structure to hold the gases that expand and to help the bread rise and become fluffy. Without gluten, baked foods tend to either crumble excessively or be dense enough to double as a lethal weapon. Using xanthan gum and combining gluten-free flours are the keys to creating gluten-free baked goods that are just as good as the real deal. I explain how to work with mixes, incorporate xanthan gum, substitute gluten-free flours, and more in the sections that follow.

Mixing it up with mixes

Cooking from scratch is terrific, and these days, especially with the help of the Real Cookbook Authors, the success rate is high, but consider using some of the incredible gluten-free mixes now available for pancakes, cookies, cakes, breads, brownies, biscuits, pizza crust, pie crust, muffins, and just about anything else you can think of. Many of the mixes are so good these days that they rival even the best home-made gluten-containing foods. They're simple to make (have the kids help!) and fill the house with that June-Cleaver-lives-here smell of freshly baked treats.

Most of the mixes simply require an egg or egg substitute, water or milk, and oil. Many of the companies are aware of multiple food intolerances and offer casein-free, corn-free, soy-free, and other allergen-free products. You can keep it simple or jazz it up, adding your favorite ingredients and accommodating other allergies and intolerances.

The most common complaint I hear about mixes is that they're expensive — and they are. But when you consider that they're pretty much fail-proof, and when you add up the cost of some of the specialty gluten-free baking ingredients such as special flours and xanthan gum — and then on top of that you add the fact that sometimes when you bake gluten-free foods from scratch, you have some failures that you end up feeding to the dog — you realize that, at $6.50 per cookie that didn't turn out, the *dog food* is expensive, and the mix is really a good deal.

Introducing xanthan gum, the star of the dough

Boasting unique properties that enhance the consistency of foods, xanthan gum is a key ingredient in successful gluten-free baking. Basically, it holds particles of foods together, and it's the component in salad dressings, gravies, sauces, and ice creams that gives those foods a creamy, rich, smooth texture. Xanthan gum has proven to work well in gluten-free foods, providing the stretch and elasticity that gluten usually offers.

Here's a guide for how much xanthan gum to use for each cup of gluten-free flour:

- ✔ **Breads:** 1 heaping teaspoon
- ✔ **Cakes:** ½ teaspoon
- ✔ **Cookies:** ¼ teaspoon
- ✔ **Muffins:** ¾ teaspoon
- ✔ **Pizza:** 2 teaspoons

I warn you, xanthan gum is pricey. Some people use guar gum instead, usually because it's cheaper. But be aware that guar gum is high in fiber content and can have a laxative effect.

 When you're making gluten-free dough, either use nonstick loaf pans, baking sheets, and pie pans or be prepared to use lots of parchment paper, wax paper, or aluminum foil. Gluten-free dough is especially sticky.

Substituting gluten-free flours

Several gluten-free flours work well for baking, but they don't always work in a one-to-one trade. In other words, you can't just replace 1 cup of all-purpose or wheat flour with 1 cup of potato starch — at least, not for the best results.

You can play around with these substitutions to find the flavors and consistencies you like best, but the following list gives you a starting point for how you can use gluten-free flours. (**Remember:** Each substitution is instead of 1 cup of all-purpose flour, and *scant* simply means *loosely packed* or *barely*.)

- ✔ **Amaranth flour:** 1 scant cup
- ✔ **Arrowroot flour:** 1 scant cup
- ✔ **Buckwheat flour:** ⅞ cup
- ✔ **Corn flour:** 1 cup
- ✔ **Cornmeal:** ¾ cup
- ✔ **Cornstarch:** ¾ cup
- ✔ **Garbanzo bean (chickpea) flour:** ¾ cup
- ✔ **Garbanzo/fava bean blend:** 1 scant cup
- ✔ **Mesquite flour:** 1 cup
- ✔ **Millet flour:** 1 cup

- ✔ **Montina (Indian ricegrass flour):** 1 cup
- ✔ **Potato flour:** ½ cup
- ✔ **Potato starch:** ¾ cup
- ✔ **Quinoa flour:** 1 cup
- ✔ **Rice flour (white or brown):** 1 scant cup
- ✔ **Sorghum:** 1 scant cup
- ✔ **Soy flour:** ¾ cup
- ✔ **Sweet potato flour:** 1 cup
- ✔ **Sweet rice flour (glutinous or sticky rice flour; *mochiko*):** ⅞ cup
- ✔ **Tapioca flour or starch:** 1 cup
- ✔ **Teff flour:** ⅞ cup

Making your own gluten-free flour mixtures

One of the things the Real Cookbook Authors discovered in the not-so-distant past is that if you mix a variety of flours together, they produce baked goods that have a better consistency and taste. Different combinations of gluten-free flour mixtures abound, and you can experiment to find your favorite.

If you're going to be doing a lot of baking, I suggest making up a large quantity of gluten-free flour mixture and storing it in a dark, dry place. That way you have it on hand when you want to bake. You can also buy many of these gluten-free flour mixtures premade.

Following are three of the most popular basic mixes. You can use them as a one-to-one substitution for all-purpose flour.

Bette Hagman's All-Purpose Gluten-Free Flour Mixture

- 2 parts white rice flour
- ⅔ part potato starch flour
- ⅓ part tapioca flour

Gluten-Free Bean Flour Mixture

- 1 part bean flour
- 1 part brown rice flour (or 1 part white rice flour)
- 1 part cornstarch
- 1 part tapioca starch
- ¾ parts sweet rice flour

Carol Fenster's Corn Flour Blend

- 1½ cups sorghum flour
- 1½ cups potato starch or cornstarch
- 1 cup tapioca flour
- ½ cup corn flour

Baking bread the gluten-free way

Those who've attempted the sometimes taste-defying feat of experimenting with gluten-free breads know that at times the word *bread* is a euphemism for *brick* and the word *edible* is an overstatement. But never fear; help is here — whether you're a die-hard baker or a newbie in the kitchen, freshly baked, great-tasting, smell-the-kitchen-up, gluten-free bread is easier than ever to make.

Time-saving tips for the gluten-free cook

I know I tend to have a *PollyDanna* approach to the gluten-free lifestyle, but even I admit that being gluten-free sometimes takes more time and effort. That's why I thought you may appreciate some tips to save you time in your gluten-free cooking adventures.

✔ Make your gluten-free baking mixtures in advance and double the recipe. Store them in large canisters in a cool, dry, dark place, and label them well (for example, "GF bread mix" or "GF baking mix"). Remember, though, not to add the yeast until baking day. Fresh yeast comes in amber-colored, tightly sealed jars or individual packets to keep it as fresh as possible, which is best for baking.

✔ Make as much of the meal as possible gluten-free. If you have a blended family, with some members eating gluten and others eating gluten-free, making most of the meal without gluten is easier on you. This practice also makes the gluten-free family member feel more included.

✔ Save your gluten-free mistakes or stale breads because one bad batch is another meal. So the bread didn't rise, the cake crumbled, and the biscuits fell apart? Save the crumbs and use them for stuffings, casseroles, coatings, or breadcrumbs. (By the way, the easiest way to make fine crumbs is to put dry crumbs into a food processor or chopper.)

Although some gluten-free breads do taste great these days, they still taste a little different from wheat-based breads. And why does that surprise people? That's like making an apple pie but using cherries instead of apples and being surprised that it doesn't have an apple flavor. Of course gluten-free bread doesn't taste exactly like wheat bread — it doesn't have *wheat* in it!

Gluten-free breads tend to look a little different, too. In spite of great strides to make them fluffier and airier, they're still a little denser and turn out best if you make them in smaller loaves. They also don't rise as much, so the tops are sometimes flat or even concave.

 You *always* need to toast gluten-free bread. Toasting gives it a better consistency and makes it less likely to crumble. Gluten-free bread is great for grilled sandwiches because the butter and grilling process give it a crispy texture and seal the bread so it doesn't crumble.

Consider a few general bread-making tips:

- ✔ All the ingredients that you use, except water, should be at room temperature.

- ✔ The water that you mix with the yeast must be lukewarm. Too hot, and you kill the yeast. Too cold, and you don't activate it. Also, dissolve the yeast in the water before adding it to the rest of the ingredients.

- ✔ Adding extra protein in the form of eggs, egg substitutes, dry milk solids, or cottage or ricotta cheese is important for helping the yeast work.

- ✔ Vinegar, usually cider vinegar, helps the yeast work and helps the flavor of the bread emerge. Sometimes recipes call for lemon juice or a dough enhancer instead. These ingredients also act as preservatives.

- ✔ Use small loaf pans for gluten-free bread.

✔ Gluten-free bread tends to need to cook a little longer, so cover your loaf with foil for the last 15 minutes or so to keep it from burning.

✔ Wait to slice the bread until it has cooled to room temperature.

Given the choice of doing something by hand or using an efficient, easy-to-clean, made-for-the-job, tried-and-true tool to do it, I'm likely to opt for the tool. If you want to use a bread machine for your gluten-free breads, keep a few things in mind:

✔ Gluten-free bread needs only one kneading and one rising cycle. If you have a setting that allows you to do only one kneading and one rising, choose it.

✔ You really shouldn't share your bread machine with gluten-containing recipes. Getting all the residue off the beaters, pan, and other parts is nearly impossible.

✔ If you haven't bought a machine yet, buy one with strong paddles, a strong motor, and a strong fan.

✔ If your bread turns out soggy, take it out just a few minutes after baking, before the machine begins its "keep warm" cycle.

✔ Keep dry ingredients separate from wet ingredients and add them in the order the bread machine manufacturer recommends. Whisk together wet ingredients before mixing them with the dry ingredients.

✔ A few minutes after the bread machine has started, use a rubber spatula to scrape the dough off the sides of the pan and back into the dough.

If you're a glutton for punishment and choose to mix your dough by hand, keep these tips in mind:

- ✔ If you're following a recipe that calls for using a bread machine, double the amount of yeast and use a little more liquid (a couple tablespoons).

- ✔ If you're following a recipe that calls for a bread machine and specifies that you use 1 teaspoon unflavored gelatin, leave it out.

Chapter 6

Eating Away from Home

. . . .

In This Chapter

▶ Setting yourself up for success when eating out

▶ Preparing for restaurant adventures

▶ Going gluten-free on planes, trains, and more

. . . .

*F*or some people, it isn't the gluten-free diet itself that presents the biggest challenge — it's getting out of the house. Even people who've been gluten-free for years sometimes feel uncomfortable about venturing away from home. Why? Perhaps it's because when you eat out, you have no labels to read, and you're limited to the selections others provide. And for the most part, you have little control over how the cooks prepare the food.

Yet getting out is important. Life in a bubble is for oxygen molecules, not humans. Does venturing outside require extra effort on your part? Sure. Might you receive a meal contaminated with gluten? Yep. Are you going to pay $20 for a meal that would have cost $6 to make at home? Darned straight. Is it worth it? Absolutely.

The reality is that you can't always be at home in a crumb-free zone with pantries stocked with your "GF" stamp of approval. Whether you're taking clients out for lunch, enjoying a romantic dinner for two at your favorite restaurant, traveling for business, or seeing the world for pleasure, you *will* be eating out. And unless you want to pout and starve, you need to know how to safely and comfortably accommodate your gluten-free lifestyle when you're away from home. This chapter is here to help with some guidelines to keep in mind when dining out, whether you're at a social event or restaurant or you're traveling.

The Golden Rules of Going Out Gluten-Free

There's no reason to let a little food (or lack thereof) ruin a good time. Armed with these practical and emotional guidelines, you can make your social experiences as spectacular as ever:

✔ **Don't expect others to accommodate your diet.** Even the people closest to you — the ones you love the most — are going to forget or make mistakes. But they don't make mistakes because they don't care. Often the lack of gluten-free goodies at a party or other special event is just an oversight. And sometimes people think they understand the diet, but they miss some of the intricacies.

If someone does come through for you by supplying gluten-free goodies at a gathering, be gracious and thankful; he or she didn't have to make the effort to accommodate your diet yet still did.

✔ **Ask what's for dinner.** When you're gluten-free and attending a social function, asking what's for dinner won't earn you a spot on the social circuit blacklist. Just tell the host or hostess something like, "I have a dietary restriction and was wondering if it would be okay to ask you about what you're serving so I can plan accordingly." Most of the time, people are receptive to sitting down with you, discussing the menu, and accommodating your diet as best they can.

✔ **Fill up before you go.** Because you can't expect any gluten-free goodies at a party, filling up before you go is a good idea. That way you're not starved and fixated on food, and you can enjoy the party for what it's really all about: fun and friends.

If you get to a party and find lots of gluten-free goodies you can eat but you've already filled up beforehand, try not to nibble mindlessly. Beware of popping buttons!

✔ **Bring your own food.** Don't worry that toting along some food may offend the host or hostess. Just discreetly explain that you have a dietary restriction and that you thought it would be easiest to bring a few things for yourself to eat. Ask where you should put them and whether serving yourself when you get hungry is appropriate.

✔ **Bite your tongue when the person throwing the event messes up.** If you discussed your gluten-free diet with a party's host or hostess ahead of time but you get to the party only to find croissants surrounded by phyllo-filled finger foods and breaded fried stuff, don't take it out on that person. Just enjoy the party and relax. If you filled up before you arrived, you shouldn't be that hungry anyway.

✔ **Enjoy the company.** Social gatherings aren't about the food. They're about the occasion, the atmosphere, the ambiance . . . need I go on? Don't lose sight of the celebration itself and the reason people are gathering in the first place.

Making smart choices at potlucks

Potlucks are tough because lots of cooks are in the kitchen. You have no idea what's in the dishes, and even foods that look the safest could have seasonings or ingredients that turn a potluck surprise into party demise.

Your best bet at potlucks is to offer to bring something you happen to love — and that can fill you up and keep you happy throughout the party. So what if you're eating only the dish you brought? If anyone notices, you can explain. Chances are, though, people will be too busy loading up their own plates to check out what you have on yours.

Dining Out: Restaurant Realities and Rewards

A great experience at a terrific restaurant is priceless. Good company, nice ambiance, respectful service, and delicious food synergize to create a multifaceted experience that's far more than just a meal.

Being on a gluten-free diet shouldn't hold you back from going out. Sure, eating at restaurants involves some risk. You don't know for sure what ingredients are in your food, no matter how much you try to educate your server and chef. Kitchen and wait staffs are busy and can (and do) make mistakes, and cross-contamination is always an issue. But with just a little extra effort, you can help ensure that your meal is safely gluten-free and enjoy gluten-free dining as one of life's more pleasurable social experiences.

 Consider the following tips for eating out, designed to help you make your gluten-free dining experiences the best they can be:

✔ **Be pleasant and grateful.** If you're demanding, you'll put restaurant staffers on the defensive. When they accommodate your requests, be extremely grateful.

✔ **Give them just enough information.** Not too much, not too little. You may have to read the server to see whether he or she is really "getting" what you're saying.

✔ **Don't be afraid to ask for what you want.** You're paying for the meal, and you should be able to enjoy it, knowing it's safe for you to eat.

✔ **Make it clear to the server and chef that this is a serious condition.** If you have to sound alarming, do so. One of the best ways to get their attention is to say, "It's kind of like an allergy to peanuts." You know it's not *really* like an allergy to peanuts, but saying it is will get their attention.

✔ **Call ahead, if you can.** Remember to avoid busy hours. See whether they can fax or e-mail you a menu. At the same time, you can fax or e-mail them a list of ingredients you can and can't have.

✔ **Know how foods are prepared.** The more you know about traditional preparation, the better the decisions you can make when ordering.

✔ **Bring your own food.** Not only can you bring your own bread or crackers to snack on, but you can even bring food for them to cook for you. Remember to offer suggestions for how to keep your food from becoming contaminated by the rest of the food in the restaurant.

✔ **Send it back if it's not right.** Of course, I'm not suggesting you be rude, but if you receive a salad with croutons on it, don't pick out the croutons and eat the salad anyway. That's not safe! Nothing is wrong with politely saying, "Excuse me. I must have forgotten to mention that I can't have croutons on my salad. Do you

mind bringing me a new one?" Everyone knows
you mentioned it; you're just letting them off the
hook.

The next sections offer additional guidance for enjoying delicious gluten-free meals while out on the town,
including tips on which restaurants are good bets for
gluten-free options and how to talk about your dietary
restrictions with servers and chefs.

Choosing a restaurant

Don't go to Sam's All We Serve Is Pizza and whine that
you can't eat anything. You're setting yourself up for
frustration and disappointment if you choose restaurants that, by the very nature of their menu selections, aren't likely to have much (if anything) that's
gluten-free.

Instead, go to restaurants that have large and diverse
menu selections, or choose an ethnic restaurant
that's likely to have more gluten-free foods. Happy
gluten-free dining starts with choosing restaurants
that are likely to have foods on the menu that are
already gluten-free or that the kitchen staff can easily
modify.

Finding eateries with gluten-free menus

Lots of restaurants have gluten-free menus these
days — some even post them online so you can
decide where you want to go and what you want to
order before heading out the door. Some national
chains that feature online gluten-free menus include

- ✔ Bonefish Grill
- ✔ Boston Market
- ✔ Burger King
- ✔ Carrabba's Italian Grill

- ✔ Chili's Grill & Bar
- ✔ Legal Sea Foods
- ✔ McDonald's
- ✔ On the Border
- ✔ Outback Steakhouse
- ✔ PF Chang's China Bistro
- ✔ Ruby Tuesday
- ✔ Wendy's

Not to be a buzz-kill, but keep in mind that as cool as it is that restaurants feature a gluten-free menu, they can still make mistakes. Maybe they have a new chef who doesn't know about contamination issues, or a server who doesn't know it's not okay to toss croutons on the salad. The gluten-free menu should give you a good starting point for where to eat and what to order, but be sure to gently remind your server that your meal has to be prepared in a way that ensures it really *is* gluten-free.

A gluten-free menu is ultra-convenient and somewhat comforting, but remember that many items on a "regular" menu are naturally gluten-free or can easily be made without gluten. So if the restaurant you want to go to doesn't have a gluten-free menu, or if nothing on the gluten-free menu floats your boat, don't despair. You can probably still find something that's safe to eat.

Opting for restaurants that are good gluten-free bets

With any restaurant you go to, you have to check ingredients in specific dishes. Always. And, of course, food preparation is an issue due to the possibility of cross-contamination. You can either ask the workers to make your food in an uncontaminated manner or opt to eat somewhere else. But as a general rule, these types of restaurants are a good bet:

- All-you-can-eat soup and salad places
- Barbecue joints
- Breakfast houses
- Fast-food chains
- Indian restaurants
- Mexican establishments
- Mongolian barbecues
- Steak and seafood houses
- Thai/Vietnamese places

You may notice lots of ethnic options on the preceding "good bets" list. That's because many ethnic foods are naturally gluten-free. Figure out which ones you like and which of those foods are inherently gluten-free. Then you can choose a restaurant of that ethnicity and know what to order.

Pinpointing risky restaurants

You can definitely get gluten-free meals at some of the following restaurants, but in general, these places aren't going to be good bets:

- Bakeries
- Cajun spots
- Chinese restaurants
- Italian eateries
- Specialty coffee shops

Calling ahead

Don't be afraid to call a restaurant ahead of time to talk about the menu and to figure out whether the chefs can accommodate your gluten-free diet. If possible, have someone fax or e-mail you a menu so you can see what the restaurant serves that's likely to be gluten-free; then call back and discuss the ingredients with the head chef. You can also fax or e-mail the restaurant a list of safe and forbidden ingredients. Sometimes restaurants are so accommodating that if you give them enough notice, they'll get special ingredients for your meal.

 Call at the restaurant's slowest time of day (if you don't know when that is, ask). If the restaurant serves lunch, you want to catch someone after the lunch rush and before the dinner crowd — probably around 2:30 or 3:00 p.m. If the restaurant serves dinner only, call earlier than that — more like 1:00 p.m. or so.

One of the pluses of fast-food places is that they generally follow standardized guidelines, so one call to their corporate offices can answer your questions about dedicated fryers, ingredients, and even food preparation. Many chains also have Web sites that list their nutritional information and ingredients, and some even have a gluten-free menu online. If you eat at fast-food restaurants often, put the information into a small three-ring binder and keep it in your car. That way, when you're pulling into the drive-through of one of your favorite fast-food joints, you have a handy list of its gluten-free items.

Making smart menu choices

Set yourself up for success by choosing menu items that are likely to be gluten-free or that the kitchen staff can easily modify to be gluten-free. Obviously, breaded and fried items aren't going to be your best bets, although sometimes cooks can use the same meat, season it with spices, and grill it instead.

So do you order the beer-battered fish? Not a good choice. The teriyaki pork stir-fry? Nope. Fried chicken? Probably not. Grilled chicken? There you go! Grilled fish or steak? Sure! Of course, you still may need to ask a few questions, but at least you're on the right track.

 Gluten-free ordering at a restaurant is a four-step process:

1. **Find the foods on the menu that are already likely to be gluten-free or could easily be modified to be gluten-free.**

2. **Choose the item(s) you want.**

3. **Ask about ingredients and food-preparation methods.**

4. **Make sure you've made your order clear and offered suggestions for how to season and prepare your meal.**

 Do a bit of research on food preparation. The more you know about how foods are usually prepared, the easier ordering is. For instance, you should know that restaurants, especially Cajun restaurants, often boil seafood in beer. And the "crab" you find in sushi is usually a mixture of fish and wheat flour.

Talking with the staff: Ask and ye shall receive

Don't be afraid to ask for what you want. People ask for special considerations at restaurants all the time, even when they don't have dietary restrictions. If you feel that the server isn't getting it, ask to talk with the chef (be tactful about it, though). Asking for special considerations for your meal isn't rude — especially when your health depends on it.

Sometimes you need to give the server or chef lots of detail, but for the most part, you should keep explanations as simple as possible and work your way into detail if you need to. You may be surprised at how little you need to say.

Of course, you've already chosen a restaurant that's likely to have gluten-free items and you've picked some items on the menu that look like they may be gluten-free or could be modified to be gluten-free. So at this point, you're ready to order. You may say something like this: "I'm on a gluten-free diet and have some special considerations I'm hoping you can help me with."

You're likely to find that the staff is very receptive. I start right in with the words *gluten-free* because awareness is spreading, and these days when you explain that you need a gluten-free meal, your server is likely to respond with, "Oh, really? Do you have a gluten intolerance like celiac disease?" At this point, you feel like that server is your new best friend, and you know your special order is in good hands. The kitchen crew will probably be on board, too. Today's chefs learn about the gluten-free diet in culinary schools, and they love to put their skills and knowledge to work to please a customer.

Assume, though, that the server doesn't seem to know anything about the gluten-free diet and simply shrugs his or her shoulders. At this point, the situation requires some explanation — but not too much. You don't want to overwhelm your server or relate your entire nine-year medical history. You do, however, need to get your server's attention. Say something like this: "I have a very severe reaction to gluten. Gluten is in wheat, rye, and barley. I also avoid oats."

Letting restaurant cards speak for you

Restaurant cards are small cards that explain the basics of the gluten-free dietary guidelines that you can give to a server or chef. Basically, a restaurant card says something like this:

> I have a severe reaction to gluten and am on a strict gluten-free diet. Thank you for working with me to prepare a meal I can safely enjoy.

> I *cannot* eat wheat, rye, barley, or their derivatives. These include kamut, spelt, durum, semolina, bulgur, triticale, and malt. I also avoid oats. Foods and ingredients I need to avoid include croutons, bread, breadings, flour, soy sauce, orzo, buns and rolls, brown rice syrup, and malt vinegar.

> I *can* eat rice, corn, potatoes, tapioca, soy, beans, amaranth, arrowroot, buckwheat, quinoa, millet, teff, and nut flours. I can also eat vinegar (except malt vinegar) and distilled alcohols.

> If you have any questions, please ask me. Thank you for working with me on this! Know that you have given me the opportunity to relax and enjoy my meal; I appreciate that very much.

If you make your own card, laminate it because it's likely to get covered in food when the chef handles it. I like to make up several of these cards and leave them behind with the chef for other patrons he or she may have in the future.

The words *severe reaction* are alarm words that, in the restaurant owner's mind, are a euphemism for *lawsuit waiting to happen*. Not that you would sue — I hope you wouldn't. But ears perk up when you use the words, and that's a good thing. Restaurant workers and management then pay closer attention.

At this point, you can make specific suggestions for how the cooks could prepare the item you want to be gluten-free (or you can hand over your restaurant card; see the nearby sidebar). Don't be afraid of overstressing the importance and the details involved.

If the server just doesn't seem to be getting it or seems unwilling to work with you, ask to talk with the chef. This request isn't a big deal. People are so afraid to ask to talk to the chef, but chefs often love to mingle with the guests and are really interested in the gluten-free diet.

Having restaurants cook the food you bring

Many restaurants allow you to bring in your own food, and they may warm it or even cook it for you. If you do this, be aware of how they normally cook their food because you probably need to watch out for some contamination concerns.

For instance, most pizza places use convection ovens that blow the flour all around. If you bring a pizza crust and ask them to use their toppings and cook it, you have to be sure their toppings aren't contaminated (they often are). Then you have to make sure they wrap the pizza securely in aluminum foil before warming it in the oven — otherwise, your gluten-free pizza goes into a pizza oven that's blowing flour all over. Same goes for bringing a premade gluten-free pizza with you; make sure it's wrapped carefully before asking the restaurant to warm it for you.

Pasta places often allow you to bring gluten-free pastas and cook them for you. Be sure to remind the workers to use a clean pot, clean water, clean utensils, and a clean colander before they make your gluten-free pasta.

Note: Restaurants don't usually charge extra to warm or prepare meals you bring yourself, but you should ask to be sure.

 I hope I'm not stating the obvious, but you probably should ask the restaurant to prepare your food only if you're actually buying some of theirs. A group of four, each of whom has brought his own meal in, won't win any popularity contests. But if one person in a group of four brings his meal, it's not usually a problem.

Remembering the art of healthy tipping

I don't take tipping lightly. When people accommodate your gluten-free diet and give you the peace of mind that helps you enjoy the multidimensional, multisensational experience of dining out, you should express your gratitude. If they've done it with an eager-to-please attitude, showing your appreciation is even more important.

 The number of people going gluten-free is skyrocketing. Every server you talk to, every chef you inform, and every tip you leave will better the future for everyone going gluten-free today, tomorrow, and beyond.

The Incredible, Edible Journey: It's Travel Time!

Whether you're getting away for business or pleasure, nearly all people find themselves leaving home from time to time. You don't have to limit or, worse yet, give up traveling because you're on a gluten-free diet. To ensure a great gluten-free adventure, the following sections present a few points that are important to know before you hit the road.

Researching your destination

Do yourself a favor and spend some time researching the area before you go on your trip. You can always find grocery stores or markets, restaurants, and fast-food places, all of which will have at least some things you can eat. But you may be able to do even better than that.

Local support groups, Internet chat sites, and list-servs may be able to steer you in the direction of gluten-free-friendly restaurants and stores, and researching what's typically available in the area can tell you how much food to bring and how much you can get while you're there.

 In doing your homework, if you find health food stores or natural foods stores in the area of your destination, call ahead and ask what they carry in the way of gluten-free specialty items. You may be surprised to find they have a huge array. If not, ask whether they would consider stocking a few items for you and let them know when you'll be arriving.

Choosing gluten-free-friendly accommodations

Where you stay can make your vacation a much more enjoyable experience. If possible, choose accommodations with a kitchen or kitchenette, like a condo or extended-stay hotel. Even a small fridge and microwave can make your trip a lot easier. That way, you can go to a local grocery store and stock up on some essentials, like fruit, milk, popcorn, deli meats, and snack items.

 If you don't have a kitchen, try to find accommodations that have a restaurant attached or that have several restaurants nearby. You can call the hotel restaurant in advance and have the staff fax or e-mail you the menu so you can discuss items you may be able to enjoy. Some restaurants may even work with you to accommodate your dietary needs during your stay.

Packing your own provisions

You may want to bring your kitchen in your suitcase. If so, then depending on where you're going and for how long, your kitchen-in-a-suitcase may include some of the following items:

- Baking mixes (pancakes, cookies, cakes, brownies, bread)
- Bread slicer or serrated knife
- Cereals that may be hard to find
- Cookies
- Crackers and snack items that may be difficult to find
- Pans to make the baked goods

✔ Pasta

✔ Pizza crusts (these sometimes need to be refrigerated)

✔ Sliced bread

✔ Toaster bags (when you pop your gluten-free bread in these, it can go in a regular toaster or oven and come out uncontaminated)

✔ Toaster or toaster oven

With any luck, the foods will survive the trip, and you'll arrive fully prepared to enjoy your gluten-free stay.

 If you don't want to lug the whole kitchen and pantry with you, consider sending your foods ahead. Either pack them up and send them in a box to your final destination or order them online and have them shipped to where you're going. Hotels and condominiums usually accept packages if you clearly mark the guest name and date of arrival on the box.

Getting there

Whether you're journeying to your destination by plane, train, automobile, or cruise ship, you need to consider the journey itself in your gluten-free plans. When you're

✔ **Flying the friendly skies:** Bring food for yourself to eat on the plane, even if you make a request for a gluten-free meal ahead of time (after all, what you're served may be something that isn't remotely close to being gluten-free). If you're hungry while in the airport, many airports have fast-food restaurants, so if you know which fast foods are gluten-free, you can always go there if you want or need to. Or you can hit up a kiosk or café that sells yogurt, fruit, and salads.

✔ **Cruising the high seas:** Cruise lines are extremely accommodating when it comes to dietary restrictions of any type. Most of the cruise lines I've looked into are very familiar with the gluten-free diet and even stock specialty items such as gluten-free breads, pastas, cookies, and baked goods. Call ahead and ask to speak with the executive chef for the cruise line you're going to be on so you can discuss the gluten-free diet with her. If the chef isn't familiar with the diet, fax or e-mail the guidelines and follow up with a phone call to discuss the specifics of what you'll want while you're on board.

✔ **Taking the train:** Your best bet in this case is to bring your own food. Why? Because the cafés on trains rarely have much that's gluten-free other than chips and maybe hot dogs (but usually they're pre-bunned). Rail lines usually don't have any restrictions about bringing your own food, so load up!

✔ **Traveling near or far by car:** Driving offers you the most flexibility, so it's often the easiest way to travel, at least in terms of accommodating your gluten-free diet. (The kids fighting and asking, "Are we there yet?" the entire way is another matter.)

Chapter 7

Ten Delectable Gluten-Free Dishes

I feel compelled to come clean at this point and advise you that I'm not a Real Cookbook Author, nor do I pretend to be one on TV. But I *do* cook, and the recipes I give you in this chapter are actual recipes that I use. Whether you're a culinary fledgling or a Martha Stewart protégé, you'll find these recipes to be simple, delicious, sometimes impressive, and most definitely gluten-free.

For even more amazing gluten-free recipes, check out *Gluten-Free Cooking For Dummies*, written by cookbook author Connie Sarros and yours truly and published by Wiley.

Versatile Blueberry Muffins

Prep time: 15 min • **Cook time:** 20–25 min • **Yield:** 6 servings

Ingredients	Directions
1 cup gluten-free flour mixture	**1** Preheat the oven to 350 degrees.
¼ teaspoon xanthan gum	**2** In a large bowl, combine the flour mixture, xanthan gum, sugar, baking powder, and cinnamon.
4 tablespoons sugar	
1 teaspoon baking powder	
½ teaspoon cinnamon	**3** Add the vanilla, eggs, oil, and milk.
2 teaspoons vanilla	
2 eggs, beaten	**4** Stir until all the batter is moistened (use a whisk to remove lumps) and fold in the blueberries.
1½ tablespoons vegetable oil	
2 teaspoons milk	**5** Pour the batter into a muffin tin lined with paper muffin cups.
½ cup blueberries	**6** Bake the muffins for 20 to 25 minutes. (Check for doneness by inserting a toothpick in the center of a muffin; if it comes out clean, the muffins are done.)

Per serving: Calories 192 (From Fat 51); Fat 6g (Saturated 1g); Cholesterol 71mg; Sodium 88mg; Carbohydrate 31g (Dietary Fiber 1g); Protein 4g.

Vary It! Instead of blueberries, consider using applesauce (I like chunks of apples, too), bananas, or other fruits.

Party Mix

Prep time: 10 min • **Cook time:** 1 hr • **Yield:** 12 servings

Ingredients	*Directions*
6 tablespoons margarine 2 tablespoons Worcestershire sauce ¾ teaspoon garlic powder 1½ teaspoons seasoned salt ½ teaspoon onion powder 4 cups Health Valley Corn Crunch-Ems! cereal 4 cups Health Valley Rice Crunch-Ems! cereal	*1* Heat the oven to 250 degrees and melt the margarine in a large roasting pan in the oven.
	2 Remove the pan from the oven and stir the Worcestershire sauce, garlic powder, seasoned salt, and onion powder into the margarine.
	3 Gradually stir in the corn and rice cereals until they're evenly coated with the margarine–seasonings mixture.
	4 Return the pan to the oven and bake the mix for 1 hour, stirring every 15 minutes.
	5 Spread the mix on paper towels to cool. Then store it in an airtight container.

Per serving: *Calories 127 (From Fat 51); Fat 6g (Saturated 1g); Cholesterol 0mg; Sodium 261mg; Carbohydrate 18g (Dietary Fiber 1g); Protein 3g.*

Vary It! Add pretzels, mixed nuts, or raisins to your party mix. You can find gluten-free pretzels by Glutano or Ener-G online or where gluten-free foods are available.

Rice Salad with Red Peppers, Garbanzo Beans, and Feta

Prep time: 15 min • **Resting time:** 1 hr • **Yield:** 6 servings

Ingredients	*Directions*
½ cup lemon juice	*1* Make the dressing by whisking together the lemon juice, garlic, olive oil, and salt and pepper.
2 teaspoons minced garlic (about 4 cloves)	
¼ cup extra-virgin olive oil	
Salt and pepper to taste	*2* In a large serving bowl, combine the rice, garbanzo beans, feta cheese, parsley, dill, green onions, and red peppers.
3 cups cooked rice, cooled to room temperature	
One 15-ounce can garbanzo beans (chickpeas), drained	*3* Pour the dressing over the rice mixture, mix well, and let the salad sit at least an hour before serving (either cold or at room temperature).
1 cup finely diced feta cheese	
½ cup chopped fresh parsley	
¼ cup chopped fresh dill	
4 green onions, washed, ends removed, thinly sliced	
½ cup roasted red peppers	

Per serving: Calories 308 (From Fat 137); Fat 15g (Saturated 5g); Cholesterol 22mg; Sodium 561mg; Carbohydrate 35g (Dietary Fiber 3g); Protein 8g.

Spicy Chicken Curry

Prep time: 20 min • **Cook time:** 25 min • **Yield:** 4 servings

Ingredients	*Directions*
1 pound boneless, skinless chicken breasts, cut into 1-inch cubes	*1* Rinse the chicken pieces, pat them dry, and set aside.
2 onions, diced	*2* In a large skillet over medium heat, sauté the onions and chiles in the olive oil until the onions turn golden brown.
One 4-ounce can chopped green chile peppers	
4 tablespoons olive oil	*3* Add the ginger-garlic paste and continue to sauté.
2 tablespoons ginger-garlic paste blend (OR 1 tablespoon of minced garlic and 1 tablespoon of minced ginger)	*4* Add the chicken pieces and stir.
2 tablespoons chili powder	*5* When everything is well mixed together, add the chili powder and the coconut milk.
2 cups coconut milk (regular or light)	*6* Cover and let simmer for about 15 minutes until the chicken is cooked through.
1 tablespoon garam masala	*7* Just before serving, add the garam masala, turmeric, and salt; then stir together and serve.
1 teaspoon ground turmeric	
1 pinch salt	

Per serving: Calories 521 (From Fat 372); Fat 41g (Saturated 24g); Cholesterol 63mg; Sodium 251mg; Carbohydrate 15g (Dietary Fiber 6g); Protein 27g.

Tip: Serve over brown rice or quinoa.

Baked Lemon Mahi Mahi

Prep time: 10 min • **Cook time:** 20–30 min • **Yield:** 8 servings

Ingredients	*Directions*
Nonstick spray	*1* Preheat the oven to 375 degrees.
8 boneless, skinned mahi mahi fillets	*2* Using the nonstick spray, lightly grease two medium-sized baking dishes.
4 tablespoons lemon juice	
3 tablespoons melted butter	*3* Wash and pat dry the fillets; lay them in a single layer in the baking dishes.
½ teaspoon minced ginger	*4* Mix the lemon juice, butter, ginger, garlic, pepper, paprika, and cilantro in a small bowl; drizzle this lemon juice mixture over the fillets.
½ teaspoon minced garlic (about 1 clove)	
½ teaspoon freshly ground pepper	
¼ teaspoon paprika	*5* Place an orange slice over each fillet.
¼ cup chopped cilantro	
8 orange slices	*6* Drain and discard about ¾ of the juice from the canned pineapple and pour the crushed pineapple and remaining juice over the fillets.
One 20-ounce can crushed pineapple	
	7 Bake the fillets at 375 degrees for 20 to 30 minutes, or until the fillets are opaque.

Per serving: Calories 265 (From Fat 51); Fat 6g (Saturated 3g); Cholesterol 161mg; Sodium 187mg; Carbohydrate 14g (Dietary Fiber 1g); Protein 38g.

Black Bean Veggie Burgers

Prep time: 10 min • **Cook time:** 10 min • **Yield:** 8 servings

Ingredients	*Directions*
3 pounds cooked black beans, rinsed and drained	**1** Put the beans, onion, bell pepper, cayenne, cumin, egg substitute, quinoa, and cilantro into a food processor or blender and process the mixture until it has a consistency that you can mold into patties.
¼ cup diced onion	
½ cup diced red bell pepper	
1 teaspoon cayenne pepper	
1 teaspoon cumin	**2** Shape the mixture into eight patties.
¼ cup egg substitute	**3** Heat 1 tablespoon of olive oil in a large skillet over medium heat; add as many patties as will fit in the skillet and fry them for 2 minutes per side, turning once.
1 cup cooked quinoa	
2 tablespoons chopped cilantro	
2 tablespoons olive oil, divided	**4** Add the remaining tablespoon of oil and cook the remaining patties.
8 crisp, cold lettuce leaves	
Salsa and guacamole (if desired)	**5** Wrap each patty in a lettuce leaf, topping the burgers with salsa and guacamole.

Per serving: *Calories 303 (From Fat 43); Fat 5g (Saturated 1g); Cholesterol 0mg; Sodium 67mg; Carbohydrate 47g (Dietary Fiber 16g); Protein 19g.*

Basic Pizza Crust

Prep time: 30 min, plus rising time • **Cook time:** 25 min •
Yield: One 17-inch or two 12-inch pizza crusts (8 servings)

Ingredients	Directions
1 cup sorghum flour	**1** In a large bowl, mix the sorghum flour, tapioca flour, bean flour, rice flour, xanthan gum, salt, yeast, sugar, garlic salt, and oregano. Then add the milk, vinegar, egg, and olive oil.
1 cup tapioca flour	
½ cup bean flour	
½ cup rice flour	
1 tablespoon xanthan gum	**2** Use an electric mixer or bread machine to knead the mixture for about 3 minutes, until the dough is soft and thick. Roll the dough into a ball.
½ teaspoon salt	
1 tablespoon active dry yeast	
1 tablespoon sugar	**3** Sprinkle some rice, bean, tapioca, or sorghum flour on a cutting board, and put the dough ball on top.
⅓ teaspoon garlic salt	
⅓ teaspoon oregano	
1¼ cups warm milk	**4** Use your hands or a rolling pin to flatten the dough to the thickness that you like your crust. (Add as much flour as you need to keep the dough from sticking to the rolling pin and the cutting board.)
1 teaspoon cider vinegar	
1 egg, beaten	
2 tablespoons olive oil	
A fistful of rice, bean, tapioca, or sorghum flour, to keep the dough from sticking	**5** Leave the dough in a warm place to rise for about 1 hour.

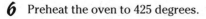

6 Preheat the oven to 425 degrees.

7 Spread the dough onto a nonstick pizza pan and use your fingers to pinch the edge and make a lip around the outside of the crust.

8 Add the sauce and toppings to the crust and bake the pizza at 425 degrees for 12 to 15 minutes, or until the cheese is melted.

Per serving: Calories 263 (From Fat 59); Fat 7g (Saturated 2g); Cholesterol 32mg; Sodium 218mg; Carbohydrate 48g (Dietary Fiber 3g); Protein 7g.

Tip: Use sauces and condiments you already have in your kitchen for a pizza sauce: gluten-free teriyaki sauce, Dijon mustard, taco sauce, ranch dressing, or barbecue sauce.

Three-Bean Pasta

Prep time: 20 min • **Yield:** 6 servings

Ingredients	*Directions*
1 pound wide gluten-free noodles, uncooked	*1* Cook the pasta according to the package directions, making sure it's *al dente* (slightly firm).
One 15-ounce can kidney beans, rinsed and drained	
One 15-ounce can chickpeas (garbanzo beans), rinsed and drained	*2* Drain and rinse the pasta under cold water.
1 cup fresh green beans, trimmed and rinsed	*3* In a large serving bowl, stir together the pasta, kidney beans, chickpeas, green beans, onion, red bell pepper, mustard, oil, vinegar, parsley, and basil.
½ cup chopped red onion	
½ cup chopped red bell pepper	
3 tablespoons Dijon mustard	*4* Toss the pasta to mix the ingredients.
2 tablespoons olive oil	
3 tablespoons red wine vinegar	
3 tablespoons chopped fresh parsley	
1 tablespoon chopped fresh basil	

Per serving: Calories 428 (From Fat 55); Fat 6g (Saturated 1g); Cholesterol 0mg; Sodium 336mg; Carbohydrate 76g (Dietary Fiber 7g); Protein 11g.

Crustless Cherry Cheesecake

Prep time: 10 min • **Cook time:** 20–30 min, plus cooling time •
Yield: 8 servings

Ingredients	*Directions*
Nonstick spray	*1* Preheat the oven to 350 degrees.
One 8-ounce package cream cheese, softened	*2* Lightly grease a 9-x-13-inch casserole dish with the non-stick spray.
½ cup sugar	
2 eggs	*3* Combine the cream cheese, sugar, eggs, lemon juice, vanilla, and gluten-free flour mixture.
2 teaspoons lemon juice	
1 teaspoon vanilla	
3 tablespoons gluten-free flour mixture	*4* Pour this mixture into the casserole dish and bake it at 350 degrees for 20 to 30 minutes. (The cheesecake is done when a toothpick inserted in the center comes out clean.)
One 21-ounce can cherry pie filling	
1 can whipped cream	
1 cup fresh cherries (for garnish)	
	5 After the cheesecake cools for at least 30 minutes, spread the cherry pie filling over it.
	6 Top the cheesecake with the whipped cream and garnish it with the fresh cherries.

Per serving: *Calories 284 (From Fat 111); Fat 12g (Saturated 7g); Cholesterol 89mg; Sodium 113mg; Carbohydrate 40g (Dietary Fiber 1g); Protein 5g.*

Easy Peanut Butter Cookies

Prep time: 5 min • **Cook time:** 20 min • **Yield:** 2 dozen cookies

Ingredients	Directions
2 eggs	*1* Preheat the oven to 350 degrees.
1 cup chunky peanut butter	*2* Beat the eggs in a medium-sized bowl.
1 cup sugar	*3* Stir the peanut butter and sugar into the eggs.
	4 Drop dollops of dough from a spoon onto the cookie sheet, about 2 inches apart, and use the back side of a fork to press them flat.
	5 Bake the cookies for 10 to 12 minutes, or until the cookies spring back a little when you poke them.

Per serving: Calories 203 (From Fat 106); Fat 12g (Saturated 3g); Cholesterol 35mg; Sodium 110mg; Carbohydrate 21g (Dietary Fiber 1g); Protein 6g.

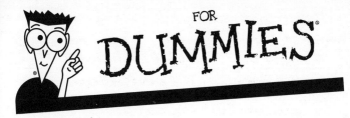
FOR DUMMIES®

What makes **For Dummies** *Health titles so popular?*

Whenever a condition is diagnosed, people need fast, easy-to-understand answers.

Readers get the essential information on treatments, medications, and lifestyle changes. They'll also find out how to begin and maintain an exercise program and stick to healthy eating habits.

Our health titles feature:

- Expert authors with excellent credentials. In fact – many of our authors still work daily in the medical profession

- Content that can be used by both the patient and caregiver

- Local editions where applicable

- A comprehensive approach to treating or managing the condition – from medications to diet and exercise

DUMMIES (FOR) *Health Titles*

Acne For Dummies
978-0-471-74698-0 • 312 pp.
$16.99 US • $21.99 CAN • £11.99 UK

AD/HD For Dummies
978-0-7645-3712-7 • 356 pp.
$19.99 US • $25.99 CAN • £13.99 UK

Alzheimer's For Dummies
978-0-7645-3899-5 • 384 pp.
$21.99 US • $31.99 CAN • £14.99 UK

**Arthritis For Dummies,
2nd Edition**
978-0-7645-7074-2 • 380 pp.
$19.99 US • $25.99 CAN • £13.99 UK

**Arthritis For Dummies,
UK Edition**
978-0-470-02582-6 • 400 pp.
£14.99 UK

Asthma For Dummies
978-0-7645-4233-6 • 380 pp.
$19.99 US • $25.99 CAN • £12.99 UK

**Asthma & Allergies For
Dummies, Australian Edition**
978-1-74031-054-3 • 272 pp.
$39.95 AUS

**Back Pain Remedies For
Dummies**
978-0-7645-5132-1 • 384 pp.
$19.99 US • $25.99 CAN • £14.99 UK

Breast Cancer For Dummies
978-0-7645-2482-0 • 384 pp.
$21.99 US • $28.99 CAN • £15.50 UK

**Breast Cancer For Dummies,
Australian Edition**
978-1-74031-143-4 • 376 pp.
$39.95 AUS

**The Calorie Counter For
Dummies**
978-0-470-56834-7 • 448 pp.
$7.99 US • $9.99 CAN • £5.99 UK

**The Calorie Counter Journal
For Dummies**
978-0-470-63998-6 • 448 pp.
$12.99 US • £12.99 UK

Celiac Disease For Dummies
978-0-470-16036-7 • 384 pp.
$19.99 US • $23.99 CAN

**Chemotherapy and
Radiation For Dummies**
978-0-7645-7832-8 • 380 pp.
$21.99 US • $28.99 CAN • £13.99 UK

**Chronic Fatigue Syndrome
For Dummies**
978-0-470-11772-9 • 384 pp.
$21.99 US • $25.99 CAN • £14.99 UK

Chronic Pain For Dummies
978-0-471-75140-3 • 384 pp.
$19.99 US • $25.99 CAN • £13.99 UK

**Complementary Medicine
For Dummies, UK Edition**
978-0-470-02625-0 • 448 pp.
£15.99 UK

DUMMIES *Health Titles*

Conquering Childhood Obesity For Dummies
978-0-471-79146-1 • 338 pp.
$19.99 US • $25.99 CAN • £13.99 UK

Controlling Cholesterol For Dummies
978-0-7645-5440-7 • 360 pp.
$21.99 US • $28.99 CAN • £16.50 UK

COPD For Dummies
978-0-470-24757-0 • 338 pp.
$19.99 US • $21.99 CAN • £13.99 UK

Cosmetic Surgery For Dummies
978-0-7645-7835-9 • 382 pp.
$21.99 US • $30.99 CAN • £14.99 UK

Diabetes Cookbook For Dummies, 3rd Edition
978-0-470-53644-5 • 392 pp.
$19.99 US • $23.99 CAN

Diabetes Cookbook For Dummies, UK Edition
978-0-470-51219-7 • 384 pp.
£15.99 UK

Diabetes For Canadians For Dummies, 2nd Edition
978-0-470-15677-3 • 408 pp.
$29.99 CAN

Diabetes For Dummies, 3rd Edition
978-0-470-27086-8 • 408 pp.
$21.99 US

Diabetes For Dummies, 2nd Australian Edition
978-1-74031-094-9 • 544 pp.
$39.95 AUS

Diabetes For Dummies, 2nd UK Edition
978-0-470-05810-7 • 396 pp.
£15.99 UK

Eating Disorders For Dummies
978-0-470-22549-3 • 364 pp.
$19.99 US • $21.99 CAN • £13.99 UK

Endometriosis For Dummies
978-0-470-05047-7 • 362 pp.
$21.99 US • $25.99 CAN • £14.99 UK

Fertility & Infertility For Dummies, UK Edition
978-0-470-05750-6 • 384 pp.
£15.99 UK

Fibromyalgia For Dummies, 2nd Edition
978-0-470-14502-9 • 360 pp.
$21.99 US • $28.99 CAN • £16.50 UK

Food Allergies For Dummies
978-0-470-09584-3 • 384 pp.
$19.99 US • $23.99 CAN • £13.99 UK

Gluten-Free Cooking For Dummies
978-0-470-17810-2 • 342 pp.
$19.99 US • $21.99 CAN • £13.99 UK

DUMMIES *Health Titles*

The Glycemic Index Diet For Dummies
978-0-470-53870-8 • 384 pp.
$19.99 US • $23.99 CAN • £14.99 UK

Hair Loss & Replacement For Dummies
978-0-470-08787-9 • 336 pp.
$16.99 US • $18.99 CAN • £11.99 UK

Healing Foods For Dummies
978-0-7645-5198-7 • 352 pp.
$19.99 US • $27.99 CAN • £14.99 UK

Healthy Aging For Dummies
978-0-470-14975-1 • 384 pp.
$21.99 US • $25.99 CAN • £14.99 UK

The Healthy Heart Cookbook For Dummies
978-0-7645-5222-9 • 384 pp.
$19.99 US • $27.99 CAN • £14.99 UK

Heart Disease For Dummies
978-0-7645-4155-1 • 384 pp.
$19.99 US • $23.99 CAN • £12.99 UK

Heartburn & Reflux For Dummies
978-0-7645-5688-3 • 360 pp.
$19.99 US • $25.99 CAN • £13.99 UK

Herbal Remedies For Dummies
978-0-7645-5127-7 • 384 pp.
$21.99 US • $25.99 CAN • £16.50 UK

High Blood Pressure For Dummies, 2nd Edition
978-0-470-13751-2 • 360 pp.
$21.99 US • $25.99 CAN • £16.50 UK

Hypoglycemia For Dummies, 2nd Edition
978-0-470-12170-2 • 288 pp.
$16.99 US • $21.99 CAN • £12.95 UK

IBS Cookbook For Dummies
978-0-470-53072-6 • 360 pp.
$21.99 US • $25.99 CAN • £15.99 UK

IBS For Dummies
978-0-7645-9814-2 • 384 pp.
$19.99 US • $23.99 CAN • £12.99 UK

IBS For Dummies, UK Edition
978-0-470-51737-6 • 402 pp.
£15.99 UK

Infertility For Dummies
978-0-470-11518-3 • 362 pp.
$21.99 US • $25.99 CAN

Living Dairy-Free For Dummies
978-0-470-63316-8 • 384 pp.
$19.99 US • $23.99 CAN • £14.99 UK

Living Gluten-Free For Dummies, 2nd Edition
978-0-470-58589-4 • 384 pp.
$19.99 US • $23.99 CAN

DUMMIES *Health Titles*

Living Gluten-free For Dummies, Australian Edition
978-0-731-40760-6 • 200 pp.
$34.95 AUS

Living Gluten Free For Dummies, UK Edition
978-0-470-31910-9 • 384 pp.
£15.99 UK

Living With Hepatitis C For Dummies
978-0-7645-7620-1 • 312 pp.
$16.99 US • $19.99 CAN • £11.99 UK

Low-Cholesterol Cookbook For Dummies
978-0-7645-7160-2 • 384 pp.
$19.99 US • $25.99 CAN

Low-Cholesterol Cookbook For Dummies, UK Edition
978-0-470-71401-0 • 384 pp.
£15.99 UK

Macrobiotics For Dummies
978-0-470-40138-5 • 384 pp.
$19.99 US •$21.99 CAN • £13.99 UK

Managing PCOS For Dummies, UK Edition
978-0-470-05794-0 • 376 pp.
£15.99 UK

Medical Ethics For Dummies
978-0-470-87856-9• 384 pp.
$24.99 US • $29.99 CAN • £17.99 UK

Medical Terminology For Dummies
978-0-470-27965-6 • 384 pp.
$21.99 US • $23.99 CAN • £14.99 UK

Medicare Prescription Drugs For Dummies
978-0-470-27676-1 • 384 pp.
$19.99 US • $21.99 CAN • £10.99 UK

Menopause For Dummies, 2nd Edition
978-0-470-05343-0 • 384 pp.
$21.99 US • $25.99 CAN

Menopause For Dummies, Australian Edition
978-1-74031-140-3 • 363 pp.
$39.95 AUS

Menopause For Dummies, UK Edition
978-0-470-06100-8 • 384 pp.
£15.99 UK

Migraines For Dummies
978-0-7645-5485-8 • 330 pp.
$19.99 US • $25.99 CAN • £14.95 UK

Multiple Sclerosis For Dummies
978-0-470-05592-2 • 362 pp.
$21.99 US • $25.99 CAN • £14.99 UK

Obsessive Compulsive Disorder For Dummies
978-0-47029331-7 • 384 pp.
$19.99 US • $21.99 CAN • £13.99 UK

DUMMIES *FOR* *Health Titles*

Osteoporosis For Dummies
978-0-7645-7621-8 • 308 pp.
$16.99 US • $21.99 CAN • £11.99 UK

Parkinson's Disease For Dummies
978-0-470-07395-7 • 364 pp.
$19.99 US • $23.99 CAN • £13.99 UK

Prediabetes For Dummies
978-0-470-52301-8 • 384 pp.
$21.99 US • $25.99 CAN • £15.99 UK

Prostate Cancer For Dummies
978-0-7645-1974-1 • 384 pp.
$21.99 US • $28.99 CAN • £15.50 UK

Schizophrenia For Dummies
978-0-470-25927-6 • 384 pp.
$19.99 US • $21.99 CAN • £13.99 UK

Sleep Disorders For Dummies
978-0-7645-3901-5 • 375 pp.
$19.99 US • $25.99 CAN • £13.99 UK

Stem Cells For Dummies
978-0-470-25928-3 • 384 pp.
$21.99 US • $23.99 CAN • £14.99 UK

Stroke For Dummies
978-0-7645-7201-2 • 354 pp.
$19.99 US • $25.99 CAN • £13.99 UK

Thyroid For Dummies, 2nd Edition
978-0-471-78755-6 • 384 pp.
$19.99 US • $23.99 CAN

Thyroid For Dummies, UK Edition
978-0-470-03172-8 • 320 pp.
£15.99 UK

Treating Your Back & Neck Pain For Dummies, UK Edition
978-0-470-03599-3 • 384 pp.
£14.99 UK

Type 1 Diabetes For Dummies
978-0-470-17811-9 • 360 pp.
$21.99 US • $23.99 CAN • £14.99 UK

Understanding Autism For Dummies
978-0-7645-2547-6 • 365 pp.
$19.99 US • $23.99 CAN • £13.99 UK

Understanding Prescription Drugs For Canadians For Dummies
978-0-470-83835-8 • 384 pp.
$24.99 CAN

Vitamin D For Dummies
978-0-470-89175-9 • 288 pp.
$16.99 US • $19.99 CAN • £13.99 UK

Vitamins For Dummies
978-0-7645-5179-6 • 360 pp.
$21.99 US • $25.99 CAN • £18.99 UK

Look for these titles wherever books are sold.